D1334427

NOV 27 2017

WITHDRAWN

UNIVERSITY

MICHIGAN STATE UNIVERSITY

OVERDUE FINES:
25¢ per day per item

RETURNING LIBRARY MATERIALS:

to remove
records

The
Silent Disease:
HYPERTENSION

Other books by the same author

The Laboratory of the Body

The Family Book of Preventive Medicine
  with Benjamin F. Miller, M.D.

How Long Will You Live?

Freedom from Heart Attacks
  with Benjamin F. Miller, M.D.

Your Heart: Complete Information for the Family
  with William Likoff, M.D., and Bernard Segal, M.D.

Adult Physical Fitness Manual, President's Council on Physical
  Fitness

The
Silent Disease:
Hypertension

Lawrence Galton,

Introduction by
Frank A. Finnerty, Jr., M.D.
Chief, Cardiovascular Research
D.C. General Hospital

CROWN PUBLISHERS, INC., NEW YORK

© 1973 by Lawrence Galton

All rights reserved. No part of this book may be reproduced or utilized in any form or by any means, electronic or mechanical, including photocopying, recording, or by any information storage and retrieval system, without permission in writing from the Publisher. Inquiries should be addressed to Crown Publishers, Inc., 419 Park Avenue South, New York, N.Y. 10016

Library of Congress Catalog Card Number: 72-96654

ISBN: 0-517-503573

Printed in the United States of America
Published simultaneously in Canada
by General Publishing Company Limited
Second Printing, May, 1973

Contents

Author's Preface

I am a hypertensive.

But even beyond the personal reason, hypertension has special meaning for me.

In many years as a medical writer and editor, I have been impressed with what medical science has become able to do to remedy the effects of many diseases.

I have watched stroke patients being pulled back from death and then later rescued, by tremendous effort, from total helplessness. I have witnessed many heart operations: the removal of useless, dead areas of heart destroyed by heart attacks; implantations of chest arteries into the heart, and by-passes of diseased heart-feeding arteries, with veins taken from elsewhere in the body, in efforts, thus far promisingly successful, to get more blood to deprived hearts.

These are wonderful achievements—as far as they go.

But they cannot go very far to solve the problem of our modern plagues. They may help a few thousand people yearly. But heart disease, heart attacks, and strokes affect millions of people yearly, most very prematurely.

The best hope for conquering any serious, widespread disease lies not in treating it but in preventing it.

It has always been that way.

Consider the once great killers. If, today, the same death rates for them prevailed as in 1900, almost 400,000 people in this country would lose their lives to tuberculosis, almost 300,000 to gastroenteritis, 80,000 to diphtheria, and 55,000 to polio—but now the annual toll for all four combined is less than 10,000.

And nearly all of that gain—and of the gain against other ex-killers, including smallpox, typhoid fever, and plague—has come about not as the result of using antibiotics and other wonder drugs, which have done some good, but as the result of preventive measures, which have done the most good, and have included improvements in sanitation and nutrition, immunization procedures, and early diagnosis.

Today, finally—much more than most people may yet have come to realize—we have an opportunity, through hypertension, to make striking, immediately practical preventive inroads on strokes, heart disease, kidney failure, loss of vision, and perhaps even on some of the most bothersome aspects of aging.

For in all of these, hypertension is a factor, a most important factor.

To no small extent, strokes, heart disease, and the other serious problems represent the *complications* of hypertension. They are, in effect, results of uncontrolled high blood pressure.

And high blood pressure is widespread.

Do you have it?

Quite possibly. Twenty-four million Americans have it. It may be present at any age, silently, producing no symptoms at all.

Is it controllable? Almost invariably—and, very often, simply.

Yet, more often than not, hypertension is not being controlled in the great majority who have it.

The hypertension story needs telling, the whole of it, the good and the bad: the recent discoveries about the critical importance of even mild to moderate elevations of blood pressure; the stealth and subtlety of hypertension, and the many myths and misconceptions about who gets it, and why, and when; the effectiveness of treatment and exactly what treatment involves; and the striking new evidence of the "vaccination-like" effect of effective hypertension control, of its ability to significantly minimize the risk of early death or disability from our modern plagues.

And, aiming to tell that story, this book is addressed to all those who need to know, and may benefit from knowing:

• Those who may have hypertension without realizing it

- Those who may be particularly predisposed to it
- Those who are aware of their hypertension but have neglected to seek treatment or, having started treatment, abandoned it because of a typical rationalization: "Why bother; I have no symptoms; I feel fine."
- Those who have thought about the need for getting a checkup for hypertension
- Those just tested and about to start treatment
- And those being treated and eager for more information, more detail, about hypertension than any physician can possibly find time to provide

If this book serves its purpose well, it will be because of the help I have had from many of the scores of distinguished physicians and investigators whose research and clinical trials have established the importance of hypertension and led to the development of effective antihypertension measures.

Over the years, in interviews in their laboratories and offices, many have patiently given me insights. I have made use of what they personally imparted. I have also made extensive use of their published research findings and medical reports—and those, too, of many others whom I have not had the opportunity to talk with personally.

For lack of space, I cannot list here all the individuals—and organizations—to whom I am indebted.

But I must mention at least a few, without assigning to them any responsibility for any inadequacies in this book:

The American Heart Association
The National Heart and Lung Institute; its director, Dr. Theodore Cooper; and Dr. Gerald Payne, Project Officer for the Institute's Hypertension Detection and Follow-Up Program
Dr. Marc J. Musser, Chief Medical Director, Department of Medicine and Surgery, Veterans Administration
Dr. Edward D. Freis, Chief, Antihypertension Clinic, Veterans Administration Hospital, Washington, D.C.
Dr. Joseph A. Wilber, Georgia Department of Public Health
Dr. Frank A. Finnerty, Jr., Chief, Cardiovascular Research, Georgetown University Division D.C. General Hospital

Dr. Edward Kass, Director, Channing Laboratory, Boston City Hospital

Dr. Jeremiah Stamler, Professor and Chairman Department of Community Health, Northwestern University Medical School

Dr. Joseph Cimino, Commissioner of Health, New York City

Dr. Irvine H. Page, Editor, *Modern Medicine*

Dr. Lewis K. Dahl, Brookhaven National Laboratory

Dr. William B. Kannel, Director, The Framingham Study

Dr. Harriet P. Dustan, The Cleveland Clinic

Dr. John Laragh, Presbyterian Hospital, New York

Dr. Melvin Kahn, Mount Sinai Hospital, New York

Dr. Benjamin F. Miller, University of Pennsylvania

Introduction

This is a book about a strange yet *extremely* common disease. Hypertension (high blood pressure) is *the* major health challenge in America today—it is the greatest single cause of death. More than 24 million people in this country have it—and, what makes it worse, fewer than half of them know they have it. And it isn't reserved only for certain types—the nervous, red-faced apoplectic. It affects men, women, and children of every national origin, and there are usually no symptoms.

But just finding the hypertensives—the millions of unsuspecting people whose health and life expectancy are so vulnerable—is only one part of the challenge. Knowing you have high blood pressure solves nothing. Treatment for patients who "feel fine" is *the* message that we must get across. More and more doctors now recognize this.

There is also the dropout problem. Patients, especially those with elevated pressure but without symptoms, will not remain in treatment unless they are strongly motivated. Such motivation can come only from a good doctor-patient relationship. This is as true in the clinic as in private practice. Unfortunately, many clinics are set up basically for traditional medical care—disease dominated, not patient oriented, and not organized for preventive efforts. Where there is no attempt to provide personal care and to foster a close doctor-patient relationship, the dropout rate is very high.

When, recently, a sociologist and I examined the reason for the high dropout rate in clinics in inner-city Washington, D.C., we found that patients failed to return not because they were stupid or insensitive to what high blood pressure might do to them, but because they were treated like cattle —they waited an average of 4½ hours before seeing a doctor.

The average time spent with the doctor was 7 minutes; they frequently were examined by a different doctor on each visit, which prevented any explanation of their disease or the establishment of a close doctor-patient relationship. It is hardly any wonder that they stopped treatment after a few such experiences. Unfortunately, their next contact with medical care all too frequently would be in the emergency room because of a stroke.

Several years ago, our hypertension clinic at DC General Hospital in Washington was reorganized on the basis of our findings—with emphasis on personal relationships and a meaningful appointment system—and our dropout rate fell from 42 percent to 8 percent.

The government has already started to attack hypertension. The U.S. Department of Health, Education and Welfare has launched a National Hypertension Information Program—an unprecedented cooperative effort involving all health forces of the government (National Institutes of Health, the Food and Drug Administration, Health Services and Mental Health Administration), combined with the American Medical Association and organized medicine, and with industry and insurance and pharmaceutical companies, to fight one disease. The main thrust of this program will be to make every citizen aware of the frequency of high blood pressure and its complications, what can be done about it, and how to take advantage of existing facilities—underscoring even to all doctors that strokes, kidney failure, and heart failure are all preventable complications of high blood pressure.

This is precisely (and more) the achievement of Lawrence Galton's authoritative book. Here are all the facts any good, concerned doctor treating or testing for hypertension would dearly love to have the time to give you and to repeat as often as necessary. Galton expresses himself in clear, layman's language—citing the conditions that are most susceptible to hypertension and how you can help eliminate or avoid them. He explains just what hypertension is and how you can know positively whether or not you have it, and how advanced it is or if it just needs watching so that it can be treated before complications set in. He also explains what to expect in treatment and how effective that treatment in your case can be. And, most important, if you are hypertensive, even mildly, he tells you what you need to know to remain motivated so that treatment can be kept simple and effective and thereby enable you to live an absolutely normal life.

Lawrence Galton has provided the tools for us all to join the battle against the silent disease.

—Frank A. Finnerty, Jr., M.D.
Chief, Cardiovascular Research, D.C. General Hospital
Professor of Medicine, Georgetown University

1

The Challenge

One minute he was walking along seemingly in the best of health. The next he was on the ground, clutching his chest. When they got him to the hospital, he was dead—at 43 years of age—a victim, according to the death certificate, of myocardial infarction: heart attack.* But the heart attack was the end cause, terminal event, result, not the real cause.

A year ago, at 49, he had a heart attack in his office—serious but not overwhelming. He was seated at his desk when the oppressive squeezing pressure beneath his chest bone came, and he tried to stand up, but his legs gave way. His secretary, who happened to walk in that moment, called an emergency number. One of those shiny new, expensive, and still uncommon, coronary care ambulances—virtually a hospital coronary care unit on wheels—got to him quickly.

He doesn't remember what happened next. Two minutes after he was aboard the ambulance, as the telemetry equipment flashed his electrocardiogram and vital signs to the hospital and the ambulance attendants worked over him, his heart fibrillated, shivered, stopped pumping blood. That was attended to at once; electrodes on his chest shocked the heart back to normal rhythm. When he came to, he was in the hospital's coronary care unit, enmeshed in wires and tubes. For the next week, he was electronically monitored and watched around the clock by specially trained personnel.

He recovered. After several weeks he was out of the hospital. His bill: more than $4,200. But he is with his fam-

* This is a typical, not actual, case history occurring nationwide, as are several other histories in this book if not otherwise identified.

ily again, back at work, one of the fortunate ones. The hospital case records show the diagnosis: myocardial infarction.

But once again, the heart attack was not the prime cause, only a near-terminal event.

Until she sat down to dinner that night, she had always considered herself healthy. But suddenly, at the table, she became dizzy and slightly confused. Her arm felt weak when she tried to lift a fork; her words blurred slightly when she tried to talk. In a few minutes, she was fine again. "The cocktails?" her children queried jokingly. But it wasn't the cocktails. Like hundreds of thousands of Americans each year, she had experienced a "little stroke." Over the next months, she experienced other little strokes—manifested by brief stomach upsets, fleeting moments of vertigo and numbness.

Then, she woke up one morning, one hand numb and awkward. Her coffee cup slipped from her hand at breakfast, and within thirty minutes one of her legs was paralyzed. A big stroke! If she is lucky, she will survive it; if she is very lucky, she may regain at least a reasonable measure of her former ability to speak, move, live a normal life.

In Galveston, Texas, every fourth Thursday of the month, a group of people gather in the Caduceus Room on the campus of the University of Texas Medical Center. They range in age from the early twenties to the seventies. Many of them are partly paralyzed and others have experienced a loss of speech.

At 7:30 P.M., the club president, whose philosophy is that "The world is a wonderful place," calls the meeting to order. He is 40, had his near-fatal stroke at the age of 32, worked intensively to restore himself, married, and now has a 4-year-old son.

This is the Galveston Stroke Club and its members comfort each other that they are not alone. The youngest member is 23; he suffered his first stroke at the age of 15.

The members tell of accomplishments, of hopeful overcoming of some handicaps—of how one, with use of only one hand, made three desk pen sets from marble; of how another learned to walk again with the use of leg braces and cane and now teaches Sunday school and visits other handicapped people who are "worse off" than she.

Of the club meetings, Dr. John Derrick, professor and chief of thoracic surgery at the University of Texas Medical Center, says: "They can make you cry and laugh. It is very moving to see such people helping each other with their problems. It is encouraging and maturing."

It would, of course, be more encouraging if there were no reason for such clubs.

THE REAL CAUSE

It happens time after time—day after day—several thousand times a day.

There is the sudden terrible experience, almost always totally unexpected.

And the blame is put in vague fashion on the event, not the cause.

The cause is something else again—and, very often, it is a peculiar disease, a silent disease, a fooler of a disease, a disease that may not produce a single symptom until too late: hypertension, an elevation of blood pressure, a hard but quietly hard pounding of the blood.

The vital statistics up to now have been discouragingly poor.

Despite all the triumphs of modern medicine, once a man gets beyond young adulthood, his life expectancy is only slightly better than it was at the turn of the century.

Currently, an American male has a 20 percent probability of having a premature major coronary episode—a heart attack—before he is 60. In a large proportion of cases, the first episode is the final episode. Within three hours, 25 percent of the victims are dead. Within the first weeks, another 10 percent die. For those who recover, the outlook is not universally bright. Even those who are restored enough to go back to full-time work have five times the likelihood of dying within the next five years as do their counterparts without a history of heart disease. Death in most cases is due to a recurrent coronary episode.

More than a million heart attacks occur yearly in the United States alone; over 600,000 coronary heart disease deaths are recorded every year, making it the most important cause of death. Coronary heart disease is also the most important cause of disability in the prime of life. Ten years ago, a presidential commission estimated the direct costs of heart disease at over $2 billion plus indirect costs of $28 billion. Today total costs may well exceed $50 billion.

At least another two million Americans are stroke victims. In 1960, 200,000 deaths were attributed to strokes, but according to present studies at Johns Hopkins the annual death toll may be double that.

In addition to the cost in lives, strokes bring great personal, social, and financial problems. Stroke patients occupy more hospital and nursing beds and make more use of social welfare services than cancer and accident victims combined.

WOMEN AND THE YOUNG, TOO

Typically, in 1967, there were 345,154 male deaths and 227,999 female deaths from heart attacks.

So, for men, coronary heart disease is a bigger killer—at least in their earlier years.

The greatest disproportion between male and female death rates appears between the ages of 30 and 60 years. The peak years for male heart attacks are the years 55 through 59. The frequency of heart attacks begins to build up among men aged 30 to 40, but it is not until women reach menopause that the incidence for them begins to increase substantially.

For women, if a little later in life, coronary heart disease is a big killer.

For strokes, the picture is different. The stroke death rate is higher in women than in men. Of deaths officially recorded as being due to stroke in 1967, 109,113 were for women and

93,071 for men, a "favoring" of 16,042 on the feminine side.

Deaths from heart attacks and strokes occur not only among the aged. In 1967, a quarter of such victims were of "working age"—25 to 64 years old. Over 200,000 persons under 65, including some in their twenties and many more in their thirties and forties, lost their lives.

Even at the ages 25 through 29, coronary heart disease ranks among the 10 leading causes of death. By ages 40 through 44, it is the leading cause of death and continues as such through the remaining years.

WHY HYPERTENSION?

We hear much now about risk factors for heart disease and stroke.

Many factors have been identified. High levels of cholesterol in the blood and excessive dietary intake of certain types of fats; excessive weight; excessive cigarette smoking; too little exercise and physical activity; tension and stresses; heredity—all are on the list.

Hypertension is also on the list. It belongs very high on the list.

If you have any single risk factor, your chances of premature heart attack are increased. A man with a blood cholesterol of 260 or above, for example, has three times the heart attack risk of one with a cholesterol level below 200. The smoker of a pack or less of cigarettes a day has twice the risk of a nonsmoker.

But a man with only a mild elevation of blood pressure—with, for example, a measurement at systole (the moment the heart contracts) of 160—has five times the risk of one with systolic blood pressure under 120.

In addition to increasing the risk of heart attack, hypertension has been shown to increase the deadliness of a heart attack when it does occur.

A study by the Health Insurance Plan of Greater New York has shown that among men with hypertension who suffer heart attacks, the number dead within a month is twice those with normal pressure before an attack. Moreover, compared with men with normal pressure who survive a heart attack, hypertensive survivors have twice the risk of a repeat attack and more than five times the risk of dying of heart disease during the next 5 years.

The higher the blood pressure, the greater the liability. But even mild pressure elevation can cut 17 years off the life expectancy of a 35-year-old man, for example.

Of all known risk factors, hypertension is now ranked as the most significant in:

• producing atherosclerotic phenomena (hardening and clogging of heart, brain, leg, and other arteries)

• development of strokes, congestive heart failure, and kidney failure

• inducement of coronary heart disease, heart attacks, and angina pectoris (the sometimes crippling chest pain associated with poor blood circulation to the heart muscle)

Aside from its role in coronary heart disease, elevated blood pressure can produce hypertensive heart disease— enlargement of the heart and main pumping chamber—with the risk that after some years heart failure may ensue. Of the over 24 million Americans who have hypertension, over half have hypertensive heart disease, as shown by heart enlargement on X rays or by electrocardiographic evidence of enlargement of the left ventricle of the heart (the main pumping chamber).

High blood pressure is thus the biggest single causative factor in all deaths.

There is still some controversy as to the role of fats in the diet, of obesity, of smoking, of stress and other factors in producing heart attacks and strokes.

There is no controversy now about the preeminent role of hypertension.

Moreover, hypertension now is known to be a significant causative factor in kidney disease and eventual kidney failure, leading to death at worst and the need for kidney transplants at best.

Hypertension is also recognized as an important cause in the loss of vision, and there is even evidence now that uncontrolled blood pressure elevation may be responsible for some of the memory loss and other phenomena long associated with aging.

Dr. Donald P. Tucker, a Rochester, New York, eye specialist, noted in a recent issue of the *Journal of the American Medical Association:* "Each year I see patients partially blinded by complications of hypertension. Most of these patients have had periodic physical examinations, but prior to their visual insult received no therapy or work-up for previously recognized hypertension. In my practice, more patients are thus blinded by complications of systemic hypertension than by treatable ocular hypertension (glaucoma).

"These visual consequences added to the other more widely acknowledged complications of neglected hypertension, make an imperative case for conscientious care of such patients from the time the disease is first detected."

Dr. Carl Eisdorfer and his associate, Frances Wilkie, at Duke University's Center for the Study of Aging and Human Development, observed 202 men and women in their 60s and 70s over a 10-year period. Blood pressures were noted and at regular intervals each patient received a complete physical examination plus a battery of intelligence tests.

Patients who had normal blood pressures showed almost no intellectual changes at the end of 10 years; those with high blood pressure dropped almost ten points in test scores.

A SECOND CHALLENGE

Virtually every single case of hypertension—from mildest to most severe—now can be treated effectively.

Yet hypertension is one of the most neglected, possibly the most neglected, of all major health problems.

In the United States it has been estimated that half of all hypertensives are undetected, half of those who are detected go untreated, and only about half of those receiving treatment are getting adequate care.

Not infrequently, by the time a patient reaches help, high blood pressure has been at work 10 years or more, destructively attacking heart and blood vessels, paving the way for strokes, heart attacks, and other consequences.

The neglect has hardly been limited to the United States alone. At a recent international symposium on hypertension, an official of the French National Institute of Health and Medical Research reported that "by the age of 50 one man in three is suffering from abnormally high blood pressure, yet we have observed in Paris that less than 10% of those who know they are hypertensives actually receive treatment."

One critical aspect of the hypertension problem already noted is that elevated blood pressure does not necessarily produce symptoms. Indeed, symptoms are rare for mild or even moderate hypertension. If elevation of pressure is to be found early, there must be regular checkups. But too many people, free of all symptoms and in seeming good health, get no checkups.

Moreover, even those who do get checkups and are found to have hypertension may or may not, because they have no symptoms, begin treatment—and when they do begin, many quickly give up, again for lack of symptoms.

In a study in Baldwin County, Georgia, public health nurses were assigned to make house-to-house calls on a sample of the population. They checked on 3,000 people and found 630 with hypertension. Of these, 45 percent did not know they had it. But even among those who were aware of their elevated pressures, most had stopped taking medication within three months.

In a Chicago study of 4,600 industrial workers by Dr. Jeremiah Stamler of the Chicago Health Research Foundation and Northwestern University Medical School, 16 percent had hypertension; of these, 66 percent did not know it. Among those who knew, 56 percent were receiving no treatment.

An Atlanta study found that even among those with severe hypertension, almost as many as went for and continued the treatment either never went to a physician or clinic for treatment or discontinued the treatment after seeing a physician. An investigator who visited them in their homes and conducted in-depth interviews found the majority could afford treatment. But because they felt well they either did not believe or refused to believe that there was any serious problem.

CHANGING ATTITUDE OF PHYSICIANS

Another aspect of the hypertension neglect problem has been the attitudes of physicians. Until recently, many physicians were loath to get involved with anything but severe hypertension. A few years ago, Dr. Oglesby Paul, professor of medicine at Northwestern University, addressing a world congress on heart disease, noted that "the physician often evades a diagnosis of mild hypertension by recording blood pressures just below 'significant levels.' Further, he all too often evidences little or no interest in initiating screening for curable hypertension, in instructing the patient in the need for long-term care, and in following the patient with adequate regularity." Dr. Paul went on to say that this was a pity because "it is not too much to say that the diagnosis, study and treatment of mild hypertension in young and middle-aged adults constitutes one of our greatest health challenges today."

Yet physician reluctance until very recently was understandable.

For one thing, until not much more than a decade or so ago, there were very limited means for treating hypertension effectively. A few potent drugs were available, but these were not without serious side effects and were largely reserved for the most severe cases of hypertension. It would have been virtually impossible to get patients with milder hypertension, free of any symptoms, to take drugs that might likely give them symptoms for the first time. The drugs could be lifesaving in very severe hypertension but, in addition to not being practical for milder cases, there was no evidence that treatment for milder cases prevented such complications as strokes and heart and kidney failure.

But then, very quickly, came an array of new drugs suitable for use in milder cases. And then, too, in the mid-sixties, began the classic studies, most notably those of Dr. Edward

Freis and his colleagues in 17 Veterans Administration hospitals across the country—working with two groups of hypertensives (one on placebos, the other on antihypertensive medication)—which showed that effective treatment of moderate as well as severe high blood pressure could dramatically reduce deaths from complications. These were carefully planned large-scale studies, carried out by trained investigators in many hospitals. The patients were meticulously selected so that treated and untreated groups could be compared. There could be no "ifs"—no questions of other factors possibly entering in. The differences in what happened to the treated men and the untreated had to be the result of treatment, nothing else.

Scientists rarely talk in superlatives. But they call the Freis VA studies "beautiful"—in their whole planning and execution.

And it wasn't long before the significance of the studies was being recognized by the medical and scientific community.

For those studies—demonstrating that early recognition and correction of hypertension before it could damage vital organs could save countless lives yearly—Dr. Freis won one of the highest honors in American medicine, the 1971 Lasker Award.

Understandably, the proof from those studies was to bring a marked change in physician attitudes. It would be too much to say that all physicians now recognize the importance of early detection and treatment of the mildest cases of hypertension but to more and more now hypertension is becoming a problem of first-rank importance in private practice and in public health, and they see its early detection and treatment as a practical means, at last, to make inroads against the modern scourges of heart disease, stroke, and kidney failure.

A PERSONAL CHALLENGE: A SUMMARY

No matter what your age or sex, there is a risk you may have hypertension. If you don't have it now, you may develop it at any time. If you didn't have it six months or a year ago, you may have it now.

Its incidence tends to increase among older age groups. But it is common in the middle-aged and even in young adults. It is found in children.

Get fat and you can see for yourself that you are; become overstressed, and you can recognize it; smoke too much and you know it.

But you can't see or sense whether or not you may have hypertension. It may produce no symptoms at all—or symptoms easily confused with other problems.

Yet hypertension can be detected readily. There is no need to wait for a screening program to reach you. There is no test as simple for your physician to make as that for elevated blood pressure. It is quick, painless, and can be remarkably rewarding.

Hypertension—undetected and uncontrolled—is a killer. If there is some controversy about some other factors that may predispose to shortening life, there is none now about hypertension.

Hypertensives are three to five times more likely than others to have heart attacks.

The risk, for them, of crippling or fatal stroke is four times greater than for others.

Hypertension is a potent contributor to potentially deadly kidney failure.

Yet, almost invariably, once detected, hypertension can be controlled. And often, the controlling treatment is remarkably simple.

The hypertension story is one of life and death urgency —of misunderstandings and myths, of still-widespread neglect, fascinating discoveries, intensive new efforts to put those discoveries to use, and new and great hope.

2

The Indictment

As a recognized cause of trouble—of heart attacks, strokes, and kidney failure—hypertension is a Johnny-come-lately.

Ironically, as recently as the 1930s some medical men thought that elevated pressure might be a good thing. It was supposed that hardening and narrowing of the arteries came first and hypertension followed—and that the increased pressure might be the body's way of adapting the artery hardening so that blood could be forced through the diseased vessels. On that basis, it was thought that lowering pressure might have dire consequences because of blood deprivation to the brain and other vital organs.

In any case, to treat or not to treat was largely an academic question. There was no effective treatment. The first indication that hypertension could be controlled—and that it was useful to control it—came when malignant hypertension in a few patients was at least temporarily held in check by surgical sympathectomy, a nerve-cutting procedure. Malignant hypertension is relatively rare. It had been overwhelming: blood pressure zoomed up, far up, and often, within less than a year after malignant hypertension was first diagnosed, the patient was dead. Malignant hypertension was a special case.

So-called benign hypertension—a term covering all but the malignant—was thus named because it was believed to be just that: useful, not harmful, except by a handful of physicians who thought that hypertension might not be all that benign and who made some efforts to treat it. But the means at hand were almost laughable.

At a symposium on hypertension some years ago, Dr. Irvine H. Page of the Cleveland Clinic, one of the pioneering and most distinguished researchers in the field, took a look back.

"It is hard to believe," he observed, "that when several of us who are here began work on hypertension, there was no treatment for it worthy of the name. True, we had many suggested remedies, such as extract of watermelon and cucumber seeds, mistletoe and garlic; and one enterprising business man sold 'whiffless garlic.' Red meat and too much sex were forbidden! . . . About 1928, potassium thiocyanate began to be used by a few, but it caused many toxic manifestations and was more effective against headaches than as a means of lowering arterial pressure."

Dr. Page remarked: "I wonder if you recall some of the regimens that were recommended confidently in the early thirties? Treatment was, of course, supposed to be based on etiology [causes], and the causes were 'worry, fear, lead, rheumatic and other infections.' Treatment consisted of psychotherapy, careful regulation of the mode of life, well-balanced diet, baths not below 34 degrees, ovarian gland preparations, iodides, and 'the bowels to be kept free.' "

But it wasn't long afterward that evidence of the fundamental importance of hypertension to the triad of killer and crippler diseases—heart attacks, strokes, and kidney failure —was to accumulate with striking speed, and it was no coincidence that the evidence began to build as the first effective medical treatments for hypertension began to become available.

THE LORD HIGH CHANCELLOR'S
VERY STRANGE CONDITION

That understanding of hypertension's significance was so long in coming is hardly surprising. For so was any real understanding of heart attacks and the other consequences. Indeed, it was not until about 1918 that an American physician, Dr. James B. Herrick of Chicago, made the first diagnosis of a heart attack.

There was no appreciation until the twentieth century that chest pain and sudden death had anything to do with the heart. As far back as 1670, physicians had been puzzled by the strange illness of the Earl of Clarendon, England's Lord High Chancellor. Clarendon experienced chest pains so sharp he turned pale. An attack would last 15 minutes. When one of his fits came upon him, he had the "image of death" before him. And in one of the fits he dropped dead.

But it was not until late in the eighteenth century that a famous British physician, William Heberden, coined the name *angina pectoris* for the chest pain that had afflicted Clarendon. Heberden noted that the pain began with physical activity and eventually progressed until it occurred at rest as well. He could offer no treatment and although he described the symptoms of angina as they are recognized today, he did not establish that angina was related to heart disease.

Not until the end of the first decade of the twentieth century did physicians begin to relate repeated episodes of chest pain, or angina pectoris, to heart disease. At about that point, for the first time, investigators in Germany began to connect angina with something even more specific—obstruction of the coronary arteries feeding the heart muscle.

It began to seem that as the coronary arteries became diseased, their inner linings laden with deposits and their bore narrowed, the heart had a tough time doing its pumping job; it wasn't getting enough nourishment through the coronary arteries to allow it to respond to increased demands upon it when there was physical activity. As the arteries became more and more obstructed, it was difficult for the heart to meet the demands even when there was no physical activity. Angina was heart pain: the cry of the heart muscle.

It remained for Dr. Herrick of Chicago to provide the first clear account of the happening in a heart attack. His patient, a man of 55, experienced severe pain in the chest an hour after a full meal, then became nauseated, and thought he had eaten something bad. The severe chest pain lasted three hours, he became sweaty and pale, his pulse feeble, his heartbeat rapid. In less than three days, he was dead. A postmortem study of the heart showed blockage in a coronary artery. Now it appeared that when a heart-feeding artery became completely blocked because of disease, the heart muscle not only cried out; it could die.

A heart attack was considered something rare in Herrick's time. Undoubtedly, it was not rare at all. Many deaths attributed to severe indigestion in reality probably were heart attack deaths. But whether rare then or not, heart attacks are certainly no rareties now.

Sir William Osler, one of the great names in medicine, had a suspicion early in the game. In 1897, Osler wrote: "Were the problem of blood pressure solved, angina pectoris would be an open book to us."

EARLIER INKLINGS

Evidently, even several millennia ago, Chinese physicians had some insight into high blood pressure and its consequences. They even discerned some connection between salt in the diet and elevated pressure. In 2600 B.C., a classic Chinese treatise on internral medicine contained a passage noting that "if too much salt is used in food, the pulse hardens, tears make their appearance, and the complexion changes."

Ancient Chinese medical texts advocated bloodletting and acupuncture as treatment "when the blood hardens." North and South American Indians used trepanning, boring a hole in the skull. Roman, medieval Arab, and Jewish physicians used leeches for bloodletting.

The Bible contains many accounts of paralysis and sudden death—stroke incidents—which may well have been the results of elevated pressure. And it is now recognized that many celebrated people in the past—from King Charles II and his mistress Nell Gwynn to physicians and scientists such as William Harvey, Edward Jenner, Richard Bright,

and Louis Pasteur, and to modern-day statesmen including
Woodrow Wilson, Franklin D. Roosevelt, and Joseph Stalin
—died as the result of complications of severe hypertension.

THE MARE AND THE MEASUREMENT

Even the ability to accurately measure blood pressure
is a very recent development.

Although William Harvey in the early seventeenth century had described the circulation of the blood, it was left
to the Reverend Stephen Hales in 1733 to perform a classic
experiment on a horse.

"In December," Hales wrote, "I caused a mare to be tied
down alive on her back; she was 14 hands high, and about
14 years of age, had a fistula on her withers, was neither very
lean nor yet lusty; having laid open the left crural artery
about 3 inches from her belly, I inserted into it a brass pipe
whose bore was ⅙ of an inch in diameter; and to that, by
means of another brass pipe which was fitly adapted to it, I
fixed a glass tube, of nearly the same diameter, which was 9
feet in length: then untying the ligature on the artery, the
blood rose in the tube 8 feet 3 inches perpendicular above
the level of the left ventricle of the heart: but it did not
attain to its full height at once; it rushed up about half way
in an instant, and afterward, gradually at each pulse, 12, 8,
6, 4, 2, and sometimes 1 inch; when it was at its full height,
it would rise and fall at and after each pulse 2, 3 or 4
inches."

Still, it was almost another hundred years before Jean
Leonard-Marie Poiseuille, a medical student in Paris,
thought of connecting a mercury-filled U-tube to an artery.
Because mercury is 13.6 times more dense than blood or
water, the column in the tube was raised to a much smaller
height and the indoor measurement of blood pressure became feasible. Since that time, millimeters of mercury, or
mm Hg, have been the standard units of blood pressure
measurement.

Even then, it was to be almost another 70 years before an

Italian physician reported a measuring instrument for arterial blood pressure, the sphygmomanometer, which had a rubber cuff—much as do instruments today—that could be pumped up to cut off the pulse. Finally, in 1905, a Russian physician reported a method of picking up sounds of the pulse, using a stethoscope, and about the time of World War I blood pressure measurements began to be taken much as they are today.

But it took decades after that to document the significance of hypertension.

THE CLUES

Following William Osler's suggestion of a link between chest pain and blood pressure, Dr. S. A. Levine, an American cardiologist, in 1929 wrote a classic monograph on coronary thrombosis in which he recognized that 60 percent of his 145 heart attack patients had been hypertensive. It seemed to him that elevated blood pressure "is probably the most common, single etiological [causative] factor in the development of coronary thrombosis."

Another milestone was reached in 1948 when investigators reported that they had found more than four times as many heart attack deaths occurring in young soldier patients aged 18 to 39 with elevated pressure than among those with normal pressure.

A striking array of facts about hypertension and life and death came from a massive insurance company study reported in 1959. Insurance companies had begun to collect prolonged follow-up data on persons found to have elevated blood pressure during insurance examinations. The data indicated a definite adverse effect on life expectancy. Moreover—surprisingly at that point in time—the adverse effect could be seen not only in people with severe hypertension but also in those with only modest blood pressure elevations.

In 1959, the Society of Actuaries published a monumental intercompany blood pressure study analyzing data on 4 million lives and 102,000 deaths. From the study, it was clear that blood pressures above 140/90 are abnormal at any age and lead to higher mortality.

For example, the study showed that a 45-year-old man with blood pressure of 150/90—certainly no extreme elevation—could expect to live seven fewer years than if his blood pressure were not that mildly elevated.

According to the study, there is a gradual increase with age in the frequency of elevated pressure. In the age group 15 to 19, 0.9 percent of men and 0.3 percent of women have blood pressures of 140/90 or over. By ages 30 to 39, the incidence rises to 4.6 percent for men and 2.7 percent for women. In the age group 60 to 69, it reaches 25.6 percent for men and 30.7 percent for women.

Generally, the higher the pressure, the greater the detrimental effect. Elevations such as 160/100 increase the risk of premature death by as much as 250 percent. But a most significant finding was the sharp effect of even small elevations.

For example, for a man of 35, if diastolic pressure is 85 and systolic is 142 (142/85), the mortality rate is 150 percent above average. With the same diastolic but 10 point higher systolic pressure (152/85), the mortality rate increases to 225 percent. If the diastolic is elevated to 95, then a systolic elevation to 145 (145/95) produces a mortality rate 225 percent above average, while a systolic of 152 (152/95) increases the mortality rate to 300 percent above average.

And there were yet to come the results of other kinds of investigations establishing more specifically how much of a factor hypertension is in increasing the risk of heart attacks and strokes—and still others demonstrating conclusively that the increased risk could be lessened by reducing elevated blood pressure.

THE TOWN THAT BECAME AN EXPERIMENT

Started in 1949 by the National Heart Institute, the now-famous Heart Disease Epidemiology Study in the town of

Framingham, Massachusetts, has been following closely more than 5,000 men and women. Its major objective has been to determine which of them, healthy to begin with, would develop evidence of coronary heart disease and to try to clarify the factors that led to the disease.

The study has provided significant insights into realistic risk factors while exonerating such previously suspected factors as inadequate sleep, moderate alcohol intake, and even coffee drinking.

In 1949, Framingham was representative, ethnically and sociologically, of the American population. Located 20 miles west of Boston, it had 28,000 residents (Framingham today is a thriving city of 60,000).

The study began simply, methodically. Of some 10,000 people in Framingham, then aged 30 through 59, two-thirds were picked randomly for possible participation in the study, and 4,469 agreed to participate. Of the latter, 4,393 could be included because they were then free of any indications of cardiovascular disease. Another 734 similarly healthy people then were chosen from among community leaders who had been asked originally to organize and publicize the study plan. Finally, there were 2,292 men and 2,845 women.

Detailed observations were made on each subject to determine life habits, environmental characteristics, familial traits, and other factors that might conceivably turn out to be related in any way to the development of cardiovascular disease. Every two years the subjects went through a thorough 90-minute physical examination that included electrocardiographic studies and blood pressure measurements.

Of the people participating in the study, some 800 have died, many from heart attacks or strokes. But in death as well as life they have helped to advance understanding. Through their participation, the study has made it possible to assess the risk of coronary heart disease and stroke in a healthy population long before the onset of any obvious disease symptoms.

Over the years, investigators keeping track of what happened to study participants found that overweight is a factor related to angina pectoris and sudden death. They found that smoking increases the risk of heart attack and sudden death. They found that elevated levels of cholesterol and other blood fats are associated with increased risk. They found that decreased physical activity, sedentary living, increases the coronary heart disease risk.

And they found that elevated blood pressure stood out as a prime factor in increasing risk.

Over a 14-year period, heart attacks proved to be three to five times more common in Framingham people with hypertension than in others. The risk of coronary heart disease, and its manifestations—including angina, heart attack, and sudden death—was "distinctly and impressively related" to the blood pressure level. Blood pressure elevation was found to contribute to the risk of coronary heart disease in the absence of any other conditions that could increase risk. The seriousness of elevated pressure, however, proved to be even greater if there were also high blood fat levels.

In order to reduce the coronary heart disease morbidity and mortality, a Framingham report noted, even some years ago, that "there is good reason for advocating early, vigorous and sustained control of elevated pressure at any age in both sexes."

The Framingham study also turned up striking evidence of the role of hypertension in stroke. During 14 years, stroke hit 65 of the men, 70 of the women. The risk of stroke proved to be four times as high among those who had hypertension, even though they had no hypertension symptoms, as among those with normal pressure. Out of the study came a clear indication that hypertension, even of mild degree, at any age, in either sex, is the most common and most potent precursor to strokes.

By 1968, viewing the continuing study results, Dr. Thomas R. Dawber, who had served as medical director for the investigation, concluded: "We should pay more attention now to borderline blood pressure levels. If we could keep blood pressure down it would do more good than anything else."

MORE FROM FRAMINGHAM

The Framingham study continues. And more recently from it has come another significant finding: hypertension is the principal precursor of congestive heart failure.

Congestive heart failure can be deadly.

It is not a disease in itself but rather a complex of symptoms arising from heart conditions. It means that the pumping power of the heart has been so impaired that it no longer can circulate enough blood to provide adequately for all body tissues. As the kidneys then become shortchanged of vital circulation, urine output drops because the kidneys no longer remove enough water from blood. The water retention leads to accumulation of fluid in the lungs and other tissues. This is congestive heart failure and when it is far advanced the patient is almost drowning in his own fluids.

Among those studied at Framingham, 142 died of congestive heart failure and hypertension was a common factor in 75 percent of the deaths.

The incidence of congestive heart failure was five times as great among hypertensives as among persons with normal blood pressure. Of those who developed congestive heart failure, 20 percent of the men and 14 percent of the women died within a year, and 60 percent of the men and 40 percent of the women were dead within five years. Management of congestive heart failure is improving but, the study indicates, if there is to be substantial further improvement, hypertension must be detected early and treated more vigorously than it has been up to now.

3

What Is It?
What Does It Do?
How?

Blood pressure may seem mysterious. It isn't. It is simply the force exerted against the walls of the arteries as blood flows through.

Primarily, the pressure is produced by the pumping action of the heart—and it is essential for pushing the body's five quarts of blood through the more than 60,000 miles of blood vessels in order to get the life-sustaining blood-transported oxygen and nutrients to all tissues of the body.

The body's system for regulating blood pressure is remarkable. It is so finely tuned and responsive that it can accommodate instantly to the changing circulatory demands of organs and tissues under varying conditions. For example, when we lie down less pressure is needed because there is less gravity to work against; when we stand up more pressure is needed to compensate for increased gravity force; also when we work, play, and eat; and even when we are affected by fear, anger, and other emotions.

To help understand blood pressure and how it is normally controlled—and what can happen when the controls become abnormal—let's step back for a moment for an orientating view of the whole cardiovascular, or heart and blood vessel, system.

THE PUMP, THE TREE, AND THE PRESSURE

The human heart—which is about the size of a fist and shaped like an eggplant—is a four-chambered pump. After blood has circulated through the body, it returns to the heart via the vein system. It enters a chamber on the top right side of the heart, the right atrium, and from there it moves to the lower chamber on the right side of the heart, the right ventricle. An atrium is a kind of storage chamber; a ventricle is a pumping chamber. And the right ventricle pumps the used blood to the lungs where it can be refreshed.

From the lungs, fresh, oxygen-rich, red blood moves to the atrium on the top left side of the heart and then into the left ventricle below. It is the left ventricle that pumps the blood out to be circulated through the entire body.

The vascular system, the vessels through which blood moves, is much like a tree. The system starts with the great aorta, the body's big main artery, which is about the size of a garden hose, and arises at the left ventricle.

From the aorta, various arteries branch off and go to different parts of the body—head, chest, abdomen, limbs. And from the aorta, too, branch off the coronary arteries which feed the heart muscle itself.

Although the heart is constantly receiving and pumping out blood—beating an average of 70 times a minute, 36 million times a year, more than two billion times in a lifetime, pushing out about half a cup of blood with each beat and some 300,000 tons of blood in half a century—it draws no nourishment at all from the blood passing through its chambers.

Yet the heart, being a muscle and a very hardworking one, must, like any other muscle, have nourishment. The coronary vessels provide it. There are two of them. They branch off the aorta at a point quite near where the aorta itself comes out of the heart, and they double back to cover the heart muscle. One, the right coronary artery, extends over the right and back sides of the ventricles; the other, the

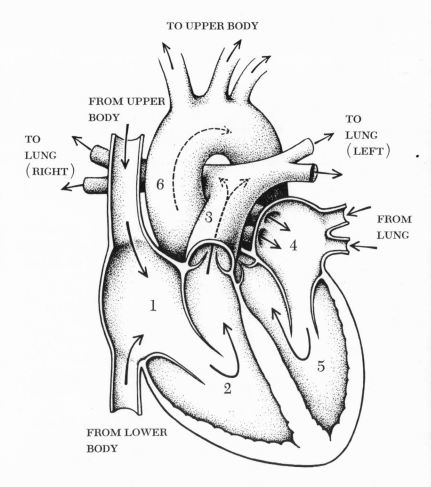

TO UPPER BODY

FROM UPPER BODY

TO LUNG (RIGHT)

TO LUNG (LEFT)

FROM LUNG

FROM LOWER BODY

The Human Heart and the Circulation. After its trip through the body, blood returns to the heart, entering the right atrium (1). From there it flows to the right ventricle below (2), which pumps it to the lungs through the pulmonary artery (3). After freshening in the lungs, the blood moves through the pulmonary vein back to the heart, now entering the left atrium (4). From there, it goes to the left ventricle below (5), which contracts to send it into the great main trunkline artery, the aorta (6), from which arteries branch off to carry supplies to all parts of the body. *Courtesy of CIBA Pharmaceutical Company.*

left coronary, supplies the left side and part of the front and the back of the heart muscle. The two coronary arteries branch into a large number of smaller arteries.

Such branching is typical of arteries all over the body. The large arteries divide, subdivide, and subdivide again, with the tiny branches ending in very small vessels called arterioles. These vessels have muscular coats and are under nervous control. The arterioles lead to capillaries, which are minute vessels with walls only a single cell thick. It is through the capillaries that the exchange of substances between blood and tissues takes place. From the capillaries, the blood then flows into tiny vessels called venules, which empty into the veins that carry blood back to the heart.

The arterioles play a particularly important part in blood flow and in determining whether blood pressure is normal or becomes elevated.

The arterioles do more than connect arteries to the capillaries. They are much like muscular tubes and they can tighten and relax. If there were no arterioles, each beat of the heart would send a surge of blood into the capillaries and into the tissues, flooding them. But the arterioles can contract and dam the blood flow so that the movement into the capillaries is in a smooth stream.

The arterioles also serve to regulate the flow of blood to where it is needed. If, for example, more blood is needed in the stomach during digestion, the arterioles in that area relax to allow more blood to flow in. At the same time, arterioles in other parts of the body may contract to minimize blood flow in those areas so more blood can move to where it is needed. This kind of activity goes on automatically. It goes on instantaneously when you get out of bed in the morning. Arterioles in the legs contract so that more blood is available to flow to the heart and brain and other organs when you stand erect.

Blood pressure depends upon arteriole activity as well as the beat of the heart. Think of the nozzle on a garden hose. When you open the nozzle after turning on the water at the faucet, the force of water pressing against the inside wall of the hose drops off. As you narrow the nozzle opening, reducing or cutting off the flow of water, pressure builds up. The arterioles act much like nozzles.

Normally, the arterioles never can be completely shut. No tissue is ever without some need for blood. Even inert parts of the body such as skin and bone require nourishment. Most of the time the arterioles are only part contracted so some blood gets through to capillaries everywhere and the arterioles in particular areas open wider when more blood is needed in those areas.

If, for any reason, arterioles throughout the blood system clamp shut or abnormally tight, pressure goes up.

MEASURING THE PRESSURE

A very simple instrument, the sphygmomanometer, is used to measure blood pressure.

You may, in fact, have made use of the principle behind it in an experiment performed in your high school laboratory days when you poured some mercury into a U-shaped glass tube. Although you poured the mercury into one end, you promptly had two columns of mercury, one in each arm of the tube, with both columns at the same height. It was simply a case of the weight of the mercury in one arm balancing the weight in the other.

But in the same experiment, if you then attached a rubber bulb and short length of tubing to one arm of the U-shaped tube and squeezed the bulb, you would see that the air pressure lowered the level of mercury in that arm and raised it in the other. If you used a scale, you could measure the height of the column as it rose or fell as air was pumped in or let out.

The sphygmomanometer works in much the same way. It consists of a column of mercury, a cloth bag to be wrapped around the arm just above the elbow, and a rubber bulb. When the bulb is pumped, the cloth bag swells with air and squeezes against the underlying artery in the arm. As air pressure in the bag increases, the flow of blood through the artery is diminished and finally stopped altogether. At the same time the mercury is forced up to a height by the air pressure.

Now, when the cone-shaped end of a stethoscope is placed just below the bag or cuff on the artery, you will hear nothing since no blood is flowing through the artery. But as air is released slowly from the cuff, the level of mercury in the column will fall, since there is less air to hold it up. With further release of air, there comes a point where the pressure of the blood pushing against the cuff is able to overcome the pressure from the cuff that has been cutting off the flow. Then as blood gets through, you can begin to hear beats through the stethoscope. At this point, the level of the column of mercury is noted. It marks the systolic blood pressure, the pressure in the artery with the beat of the heart.

As still more air is released from the cuff, the sound of blood pulsing through the artery first becomes louder but then fades. At this point, the level of the column of mercury is read again. It marks the diastolic blood pressure, the low level reached when the heart relaxes between beats and, momentarily, there is no new surge of blood from the heart into the arteries.

Since no two people are exactly alike in anything, including the force of the heartbeat and the activity of arterioles, there is a wide range of blood pressure in healthy, normal people. A systolic pressure between 100 and 140 mm Hg is considered normal; so is a diastolic pressure between 60 and 90.

It is when pressure goes above the upper limits of normal that hypertension has to be considered.

Once it was believed that hypertension should not be diagnosed until the diastolic pressure exceeded 95 (some physicians thought 100) and the systolic exceeded 160. The range between 140/90 and 160/95 was regarded as borderline. More and more physicians today, however, become concerned at any elevation beyond 140/90. They may or may not begin treatment at this point, but they do keep closer tabs on the patient's blood pressure thereafter, on guard for any further elevation.

It used to be thought, too, that there was a relationship

between age and systolic pressure and if systolic pressure equaled the sum of 100 plus the individual's age, that was normal. No longer. There is some argument over whether blood pressure should, normally, increase at all with age; it does not invariably do so. And many physicians now consider that, regardless of age, blood pressures greater than 140/90 may fall into the hypertension category.

Blood pressure varies, quite normally, at different times in the same individual. It goes up during physical exertion or emotional excitement. During sleep, pressure drops as much as 23 percent. Even brief arousal from sleep is accompanied by a rise in pressure. Usually, dreams have little effect on pressure but an occasional dream, perhaps an unpleasant one, may raise the pressure markedly.

Investigators have now noted that during sleep, hypertensive people show less of a decline in blood pressure than do normal people. Generally, while normals show drops of 21 percent for systolic and 23 percent for diastolic, hypertensives have drops of only 9 percent for systolic and 11 percent for diastolic.

Because of the quite-normal variations in pressure, especially the tendency for the pressure to go up during moments of tension or excitement, physicians do not accept any one reading above 140/90 as indicative of hypertension. They may make repeated measurements during one visit, and, very often, will repeat the measurements over the course of several visits before arriving at a diagnosis of hypertension.

3rd Sect.

BLOOD PRESSURE CONTROLS

There are important reasons why blood pressure has to be kept under control, maintained within certain limits. For example, the kidneys' work of filtering waste materials from the blood depends upon pressure, and filtration stops if pressure falls much below 60. During sleep, with the body in horizontal position, there is less effect of gravity and less pressure is needed to get blood to the brain, but pressure increases when the upright position is assumed in order to counter the gravity effect.

Pressure levels higher than the minimum needed for good functioning of the body do not necessarily produce an immediate disadvantage. But the higher the level of pressure, the greater the long-term risk of disease. If pressure rises to extremely high levels, there is even a short-term risk of failure of the heart's left ventricle because it is given so much work to do in pumping blood into the aorta and out to the body against the great pressure.

One factor in determining blood pressure is the heart's output of blood. With each beat, the heart may push out a greater or lesser amount depending upon whether, for example, you are at rest or exercising vigorously.

Blood pressure also may vary with changes in the capacity of the vessels through which blood flows, especially the tiny arterioles. Normally, the arterioles have "tone," they are slightly constricted so they respond promptly when called upon.

The word "tone" of course is familiar to athletes and sports fans. Muscles work by contraction. If they are loose and flabby, extended to their full length when relaxed, their response when called upon to contract may be somewhat sluggish. In the physically fit athlete, the muscles are slightly constricted and thus have good tone.

Actually, the relationship between the blood flow (the output of blood from the heart) and the resistance offered by the vessels is such that the blood pressure equals Flow × Resistance.

Therefore, it follows that pressure can be maintained within reasonable bounds only if resistance tends to fall whenever there is a marked increase in the output of blood from the heart.

This, in fact, takes place because of specialized groups of pressure-sensitive cells called baroreceptors. The mechanism is much like that of a thermostat used to keep temperature at a constant level in the home. The thermostat has a heat-sensitive element that breaks a circuit and turns off the furnace when temperature gets beyond a set point, then closes the circuit and starts up the furnace again when temperature falls below a set point.

The human barostat for maintaining pressure within a comfortable range is the pressure-sensitive cells within the walls of arteries. These cells, or baroreceptors, are pre-set to a narrow blood-pressure range. When pressure rises above or falls below appropriate levels, the barostat system works to bring it back within the levels.

There are baroreceptors scattered throughout the arterial system but among the most important are those in the aorta and in the carotid sinus located where the carotid artery to the head branches in the neck. The carotid sinus baroreceptors continuously watch blood pressure in the carotid artery and when changes in pressure are detected, the baroreceptors act to stabilize the pressure.

There is a story, perhaps apocryphal, of eighteenth-century French schools for young ladies that instructed their students that they must swoon at certain stories. Since swooning didn't come easily to many girls, they were taught

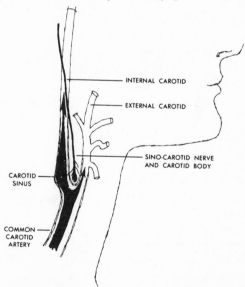

INTERNAL CAROTID

EXTERNAL CAROTID

SINO-CAROTID NERVE AND CAROTID BODY

CAROTID SINUS

COMMON CAROTID ARTERY

Carotid Baroreceptor. *Courtesy U.S. Department of Health, Education, and Welfare.*

how to manage it. All a girl had to do was to play with her necklace and, upon hearing a story calling for a swoon, push her fingers firmly into the side of her neck. With increased pressure at the side of the neck—on the carotid sinus—blood pressure falls and faintness results.

If, for example (swooning aside), during physical activity the heart increases its output of blood, the arteries are then filled with more blood and become distended. The pressure-sensitive receptors sense the distension of arterial walls and send signals through the nervous system, which cause the arterioles to relax just enough to let the greater volume of blood out of the artery system into the capillaries and tissues and thus, at once, get the blood where it is needed and maintain the blood pressure at proper level.

Let's look at the nervous system. The body has two great networks of nerves. One, the central nervous system, includes the brain. This is the system you use for voluntary control of activities. The other, the autonomic nervous system, with branches connecting to heart, blood vessels, gastrointestinal and urinary tracts, is automatic and can function without conscious thought.

The autonomic system, in fact, is made up of two opposing systems: sympathetic and parasympathetic. The sympathetic system can act when you are exercising, working hard, or worrying excessively. At such times, it can increase the heart rate or constrict blood vessels. On the other hand, the parasympathetic system can act to slow the heart rate or dilate the blood vessels. Thus, the autonomic system plays an important role in controlling blood pressure through its effects on heart and blood vessels.

Blood pressure may also be profoundly affected by certain hormones. Two in particular, norepinephrine and epinephrine, from the adrenal glands atop the kidneys, are powerful blood-vessel constrictors. Both are secreted in increased quantities during vigorous exercise and also during fright or other severe emotional stress.

Not only do many mechanisms operate in the regulation of blood pressure; they may interact.

The barostatic mechanism can regulate resistance in the

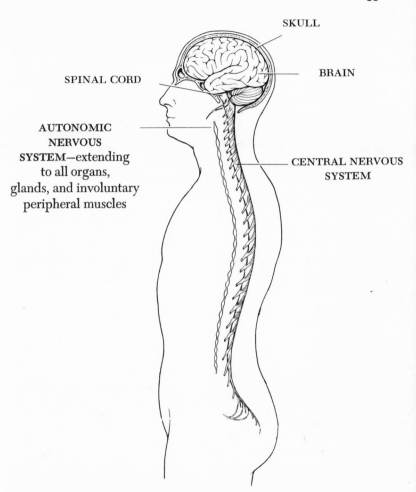

SKULL

BRAIN

SPINAL CORD

AUTONOMIC
NERVOUS
SYSTEM—extending
to all organs,
glands, and involuntary
peripheral muscles

CENTRAL NERVOUS
SYSTEM

The Two Nervous Systems (a schematic representation). The well-known central nervous system, housed within the spinal cord and also including the brain itself, connects to every part of the body by means of 43 pairs of nerves—12 cranial, the remaining 31 going to muscles throughout the body, for voluntary control. Also running along the spinal column is the autonomic nervous system. Its nerves extend to, and automatically control, glands such as sweat, salivary, liver, and pancreas; muscles such as those in the iris of the eyes, heart, stomach, intestines, bladder. The autonomic nerves also extend to and control muscles in the walls of blood vessels. *Courtesy of CIBA Pharmaceutical Company.*

arterioles by opening and closing them according to need. The center for this pressure-regulatory mechanism is located at the base of the brain where it receives signals from the baroreceptors and in turn sends out signals at once via the autonomic nervous system to the arterioles.

However, impulses from this center to the arterioles can be modified by chemical substances circulating in the blood, which may either strengthen or weaken the arterioles' response to the impulses. Chemical substances that raise blood pressure by increasing arteriole sensitivity to nervous impulses are called pressor substances; those which reduce sensitivity and lower blood pressure are depressor agents. Such pressor and depressor effects are produced by some hormones normally found in the body, by other hormones that may be turned out only under abnormal conditions, and by drugs.

Thus disturbances of pressure regulation can result if the barostat somehow is set too high or too low so that inadequate nervous impulses are sent to the arterioles. Or normal impulses may be improperly modified by the presence of chemical substances.

Disturbances of pressure regulation may be either temporary or permanent. Temporary elevation of blood pressure, for example, may occur in normal people during periods of stress, anger, and excitement, because of an excess of pressor hormones produced in the body during such periods. The hormones are produced to help mobilize body resources in such emergency periods—and they also elevate blood pressure. On the other hand, temporary falls in blood pressure may occur in normal individuals after prolonged standing as the result of fatigue of regulatory mechanisms, leading to fainting.

EFFECTS OF HYPERTENSION

Brief periods of elevation of blood pressure rarely do harm. It is when blood pressure remains elevated for extended periods that damage may result, particularly for certain major target organs: the heart, the kidneys, the brain, and the arteries.

The Hypertensive Heart

We've seen that when blood pressure is elevated, the heart must spend more energy to pump blood and that the pressure elevation stems from resistance by the arterioles to blood flow. If pressure is elevated, say, 20 percent above normal, the heart must work 20 percent harder.

To perform the increased work, the heart muscle thickens and increases in size. The heart enlarges and the enlargement is visible on X-ray pictures. The phenomenon is much like what happens when you exercise any muscle strenuously and consistently, for example, the biceps muscles in your arms; their girth increases.

For a period of time, despite the increased work load, the heart does well. It accommodates and handles the burden. But there comes a time when it tires, is unable to fully meet the strain. The result is congestive heart failure.

In heart failure, the heart does not stop beating. It continues to beat and to pump blood but its contractions are no longer as complete and effective. With each contraction or beat, less volume of blood is pumped.

There are many effects of loss of pumping efficiency or heart failure. Since less blood supply reaches the tissues of the body, muscles suffer for lack of adequate nourishment and there is muscle fatigue. Less blood supply may reach the brain and the patient may not be able to think as effectively as he once did.

There is a buildup of pressure within the heart itself. Unable to pump out blood with its old efficiency, the heart experiences increased internal pressure as its chambers dilate and become reservoirs for abnormal amounts of blood. The pressure extends backward to the lungs, which may then retain fluids—as much as several liters of fluids. From the lungs, the pressure is transmitted still further back to the veins of the body, the liver, and the legs. The liver becomes congested and enlarged; the legs swell with fluids; the neck veins become distended.

In some cases, hypertension has another effect on the heart. When a muscle increases in size, as does the hypertensive heart, the blood vessels supplying the heart do not increase in size. There is some spare capacity and up to a point it may suffice. But in some cases the burden on the heart is so great that its blood needs outdistance the spare capacity of the blood supply. As a result, there may be coronary insufficiency with chest pain (angina pectoris) or even death of some tissue in an area of heart muscle (myocardial infarction).

Thus in hypertensive heart disease, the damage can take the form of heart enlargement, with congestive heart failure or coronary insufficiency, or sometimes both.

The Kidneys

In long-continued hypertension, blood flow to the kidneys may be impaired. The arterioles there, too, are clamped down abnormally. As blood supply to the kidneys is reduced, they can no longer function at full capacity. They become less effective in ridding the body of waste products. There is a tendency for salt to be retained instead of properly excreted. Salt tends to attract water. Thus there is abnormal fluid retention and such fluid retention increases the chances for heart failure to develop.

Kidney damage from hypertension may also include gradual destruction of the tiny filtration units where urine is formed. As more and more are destroyed, kidney function deteriorates and eventually total kidney failure may follow, with uremic poisoning and death.

The Brain

In any pumping system, wear on both pump and pipelines depends upon the degree of strain. If, for example, a system is designed to take a maximum strain of 100 pounds, it will last longer if the actual strain never reaches that level. If the strain persistently goes above 100 pounds, the system eventually will deteriorate.

One form of deterioration in the blood pipelines, the arteries, is rupture, or blowout. After long periods of excessive pressure, an artery wall may become so weakened that it finally blows out. This seems to be most likely to happen in brain arteries, which are not so well embedded in firm protective surrounding tissues as are many other arteries of the body.

A brain hemorrhage, resulting from the blowout of a brain artery, is one form of cerebral vascular accident, or stroke.

In addition to hemorrhage within the brain, destroying brain substance and causing stroke, an accident may occur outside the brain (subarachnoid hemorrhage) when small blister-like outpouchings of artery walls at the base of the brain rupture and cause massive bleeding and death.

With extremely high pressure, another complication may be the swelling of brain substance, called hypertensive encephalopathy, which may produce violent headaches, brain function disturbances, and coma.

Brain arteries are also subject—as are the coronary arteries feeding the heart and other major arteries of the body—to another kind of damage from atherosclerosis, or the narrowing and clogging of arteries. When artery clogging advances to a point where circulation to a brain area is cut off, a stroke may result. There is death of the brain tissue just as there is death of heart muscle tissue when atherosclerosis finally cuts off circulation to part of the heart muscle.

And hypertension now is known to be a major factor in atherosclerosis.

HYPERTENSION AND ATHEROSCLEROSIS, AND HEART PAIN AND HEART ATTACK

The earliest visible indication of atherosclerosis is a thin line, a fatty streak, on the inside wall of an artery. It contains an accumulation of cholesterol, cholesterol compounds, and some fats. Later, as the streak grows to become the typical "plaque" of atherosclerosis, it begins to look like a collection of mush or gruel. As the plaque, or mushy deposit, continues to grow, it extends into the artery channel and begins to offer some obstruction to the free flow of blood through the artery.

Atherosclerosis can affect any artery—in the brain, in the coronary system feeding the heart, in the leg. For reasons not entirely clear, it has a particular predilection for most often doing its worst in the coronary system.

It can be many years before there is evidence of any obvious effects from coronary atherosclerosis, of the gradual buildup of plaques within the coronary arteries feeding the heart.

Actually, much of the human body is "spare" in a sense. There are "extras," so that, if necessary, we can get along with one kidney instead of two, with one lung instead of two, with even half the brain.

And in a healthy person the coronary arteries can carry much more blood to the heart than the heart normally requires. As a result, for many years, as the coronary arteries are increasingly affected by atherosclerosis, they may still be able to get enough blood to the heart muscle for ordinary purposes.

But then may come the day when the narrowing of the arteries reaches a point where there is no longer enough blood flow for any extra demand on the heart.

There have been no symptoms before. But then it happens —it may be while the victim is running to catch a bus, shoveling snow, walking to the nineteenth hole, or under great emotional stress. The heart is asked to work harder, increasing the demand on the coronary arteries to supply the heart muscle with more nourishment, but the coronaries can't supply it.

The heart is deprived and it rebels. It cries out in pain. This is angina pectoris. The victim feels as if his chest were being crushed, as if a constricting band were being drawn tighter and tighter around his chest. He may feel pain shooting into an arm, or even into his face. He stops whatever he is doing (he has to stop). Very quickly after he stops, the pain stops.

But from then on, he may experience the same attack whenever he exerts himself a bit or becomes unduly excited. But there are medications to help him. One of these is nitroglycerin. Placed under the tongue, from where it can be quickly absorbed, it often produces fast relief for an angina attack. Nitroglycerin also may help reduce the likelihood of attacks when it is taken prophylactically, that is, just before the victim engages in activities known to bring on his angina.

Angina pain can be agonizing. For some victims, it brings with it a sensation of imminent death. However, angina can be present for many years without damage to the heart muscle, provided the atherosclerosis does not progress markedly.

When does a heart attack come? It may appear if an atherosclerotic plaque roughens, provides a surface on which blood may clot, and the clot then completely obstructs a coronary artery or one of its branches. Or it may appear if the plaque bursts open and spills out so much of its material that the artery becomes blocked, with the same effect as blockage by a blood clot.

Blockage of a coronary artery or a branch deprives the heart muscle area supplied by that vessel of oxygen and nutrients. That area dies. This is a heart attack, also called a coronary occlusion or a myocardial infarction.

It is not invariably fatal. The outcome depends on how much heart muscle is affected, and the location of the affected area. If a large portion of the left ventricle, the major pumping chamber of the heart, is affected, death may follow. The heart is unable to circulate enough blood to maintain life.

If a smaller area of heart muscle, or a less vital area, is affected, life can go on. The affected area will be scarred but the rest of the heart will remain active. Sometimes the affected area will so disturb the electrical activity that governs the beating of the heart, in effect, becoming a barrier to the beat-controlling impulses, that abnormal rhythms may develop. One such rhythm, ventricular fibrillation, produces a useless quivering of the heart; it can pump no blood. Unless fibrillation is immediately corrected—electric shock applied to the chest wall may be used for the purpose—death follows quickly.

If a heart attack victim is fortunate enough to reach a modern coronary care unit, his heart can be monitored constantly with sophisticated electronic devices that often pick up the earliest signs of abnormal rhythm changes and allow them to be corrected quickly.

All of this is by no means a full account of what may happen in a heart attack. Sometimes an affected heart muscle area may balloon out like the weakened wall of an automobile tire. If it should burst, death may follow in minutes. Without bursting, the ballooning out may so interfere with the heart's pumping efficiency that surgery becomes necessary. The damaged section is removed and the remainder of the heart is sewn together—often successfully.

Another possibility is that a damaged heart wall causes the formation of a blood clot within a chamber of the heart, and pieces of the clot may break off and cause serious trouble by blocking a vital artery in a lung, kidney, or leg.

WHY ATHEROSCLEROSIS?

What provokes the buildup of deposits in the arteries? No other question has produced so much thoughtful controversy within the medical profession and so much confusion in the public mind.

It used to be thought that atherosclerosis was something that came with the years, an inevitable product of aging. It just happened and had to be accepted. But then came such findings as these: In South Africa, the Bantu are remarkably free of atherosclerosis and heart disease at any age. And in young American soldiers—some still in their teens—killed on the battlefields of Korea, autopsies showed significant atherosclerosis.

Atherosclerosis could develop very early; in some cases, as in the Bantu, it did not develop even at advanced age. It could not be that age was its cause.

At various times, various factors have been held to be *the* preeminent cause. But it is now recognized by physicians and medical investigators that atherosclerosis is not due to some one factor and nothing else—but rather stems from a variety of factors that may interact.

Modern diet, with its high levels of cholesterol and other fatty substances in many foods, has been blamed for years. Cholesterol is found in atherosclerotic plaques. Cholesterol, which is actually a natural body substance and a vital one, is produced by the liver. It plays many roles in body functions, including helping to regulate the passage of materials in and out of body cells, and is needed for the manufacture of essential hormones. Thus, up to a point, cholesterol is vital. Too much of it, however, can cause trouble.

It has been established clearly enough that some of the most widely used foods—meat and dairy products, which are high in saturated fats; eggs and organ meats, which are high in cholesterol—can, if used to excess, raise the level of cholesterol in the blood.

Obesity is another factor in atherosclerosis. It has been shown that life expectancy may be shorter for people who are markedly over ideal weight. Middle-aged men who are 20 percent overweight, for example, have two to three times the risk of fatal heart attack as men of normal weight. Obesity also carries with it a greater likelihood of elevated blood cholesterol levels—and of diabetes. And diabetes, if uncontrolled, is associated with a rise of cholesterol and other fats in the blood and with the development of atherosclerosis.

A case has been built up also against cigarette smoking (see Chapter 7). The heart attack rate in heavy cigarette smokers is two to three times as great as in nonsmokers, pipe or cigar smokers, and former cigarette smokers. Autopsy studies suggest that cigarette smoking is associated with a significant increase in atherosclerosis.

Scientific studies also show that men who lead sedentary

lives run a higher risk of heart attack than those who get regular exercise. For exercise tones the muscles, stimulates the circulation, helps keep one from becoming overweight. It tones the heart as well as other muscles, making it more efficient in performance, able to accomplish more work with less effort, much as it does other muscles. There is some evidence that exercise helps, too, by encouraging the formation of extra blood vessels—collateral vessels, as they are called—to nourish the heart and to take over, rerouting blood to the heart muscle, if a coronary vessel should become clogged. Investigators also have found evidence that exercise may help to reduce blood fat levels.

And the role of hypertension, in itself and in combination with the other factors, has come to be recognized increasingly by medical investigators though not yet by much of the public.

THE CRITICAL ROLE OF HYPERTENSION

Can hypertension foster atherosclerosis?

One indication of its cardinal role in doing so lies in the pulmonary arteries. Here, unlike in other arteries of the body, atherosclerosis is rarely found. And here blood pressure is low. The pulmonary arteries go from heart to lungs; the distance is relatively short. The pulmonary arteries end in a vast network of capillaries in the lungs which accommodate great amounts of blood and offer little resistance to blood flow. The result is that blood pressure in the pulmonary arteries is very low—as low as 35/15.

Why should the pulmonary arteries be virtually immune to fatty deposits and atherosclerosis? It is subject to all the same factors as the other arteries—the influences of diet, smoking, obesity, heredity, stress—all, that is, but one: hypertension.

Chronic hypertension fosters the development of atherosclerosis. How? One mechanism could be that increased pressure—pounding pressure over prolonged periods—damages artery linings, disrupts the normal surface, and in so doing paves the way for deposits to be formed in the damaged sites.

Many studies have shown the very large proportions of patients with heart attacks known to have high blood pressure before the attacks. In five series of men and three series of women studied, the percentages were 58, 54, 64, 57, 41, 52, 60, and 71.

In the study in Framingham, Massachusetts, a consistent correlation was found between blood pressure at the start of the study and the incidence of new coronary artery disease in the next eight years. Over that period, men and women who had normal pressure to begin with had only one-fourth the coronary disease generally expected among people of their age and sex. Those with elevated pressures to begin with had twice the expected rate of coronary disease, or eight times as much as the normotensives. And the higher the pressure the more the risk of coronary disease increased.

Investigators in one study patiently dissected and extracted the fatty deposits from various arteries of 184 consecutive patients who had died. They found a significant correlation between the amount of fat in the brain and heart arteries and the blood pressure measured during life.

At the University of Pittsburgh, Dr. Campbell Moses, now medical director of the American Heart Association, studied atherosclerosis lesions during some 500 autopsies. He found a marked increase in the incidence and severity of atherosclerosis in coronary and brain arteries in men who had been hypertensive and an even more marked increase in women who had been hypertensive.

Occasionally some hypertensive patients have been found to have hemorrhages in one eye but not in the other. In these patients, a clot has been found in the carotid artery, a major head artery—a clot in the carotid artery on the healthy eye side. The clot lowered the pressure on that side, serving to provide some protection against elevated pressure damage to the carotid artery and branches from it beyond the point of clotting. On that side, these arteries had a normal appearance and absence of disease. On the other hand, there was evidence of distinct artery disease on the side where the arteries were exposed to high pressure.

The same phenomenon has been observed in experiments with animals. Drugs have been used to produce hypertension in the animals. Investigators then have tied off one carotid artery, thereby reducing the arterial pressure on that side of the brain. In these animals, much artery disease was found associated with hypertension on the untied-off side. On the tied-off side, where there was some protection from elevated pressure, there was no artery disease.

AND STILL MORE EVIDENCE

Investigators also have worked with various animals—rats, rabbits, dogs—and have been able to show that they could produce elevated blood cholesterol levels and atherosclerosis when they fed the animals a diet high in cholesterol. But when they made the animals hypertensive, atherosclerosis developed much more rapidly and severely and often led to heart attacks.

In other experiments, hypertensive rats have been kept on a high-cholesterol diet for 120 days. But in half the rats, blood pressure was brought down to normal or near-normal levels by antihypertensive drugs. In this treated group, atherosclerosis was far less marked than in the untreated.

It is possible to take a pair of laboratory animals and link them together in such a way that their circulations cross. One member of the pair can be made hypertensive and both can be fed a high-cholesterol diet. The blood pressures will be different, but the cross circulation keeps the cholesterol level the same for both animals.

In such experiments, blood cholesterols have risen in response to the diet. They have risen in both animals. But, at sacrifice, the hypertensive animals have shown atherosclerosis and heart damage; the normotensive animals have had minimal atherosclerosis and no heart damage.

In another approach, blood cholesterol levels were compared in groups of hypertensive and normotensive rats kept on either a standard diet or a high cholesterol diet. It made no difference: hypertension increased cholesterol levels significantly whether the animals were on a standard diet or on a high cholesterol diet. Diet increased the effect of hypertension on cholesterol but diet alone had no effect.

In other animal studies, investigators have been able to show that there is a difference in the rate at which cholesterol is produced in the body in animals with normal pressure and in those with hypertension. Hypertension does something that increases the rate of cholesterol formation in the liver and in artery walls.

What such experiments have demonstrated, then, is that (1) hypertension intensifies any atherosclerosis that may stem from diet, and that drug control of the hypertension reverses this effect; (2) that hypertension increases the deposition of cholesterol in the artery wall and that this increased deposition does not depend upon increased blood cholesterol; and (3) that hypertension increases the rate of cholesterol production in the liver and the arteries.

4

Do You Have It?
Myths, Facts, Symptoms,
and the Lack of Them

Bill B. is a 6'1", big, brawny, 39-year-old airline pilot. There is nothing about him visibly to suggest that anything could be wrong with him. But airline policy requires that he get regular checkups. And so, feeling full of health, he marched in for his latest not long ago, greeting the physician good-humoredly: "This is really a waste of your time. I couldn't feel better."

But after unsnapping the blood pressure cuff from Bill's arm for the second time, having taken an earlier reading almost at the beginning of the checkup, the doctor suggested a return visit in a week. And during that visit, after taking blood pressure measurements several times, the doctor said quietly: "It's nothing much, Bill—just slightly above normal. But we're going to do something about it."

Bill is one of the lucky ones.

In matters of health there are often misconceptions. About hypertension, there are many. It is commonly believed that hypertension is a disease of the aged, certainly not a frequent one among the young. It is also commonly supposed that when it occurs, hypertension produces unmistakable effects such as poundings in the head and palpitations of the heart. It is even commonly supposed that it's possible to tell a hypertensive person by appearance, by a typically red-faced, vein-engorged appearance.

Just about every common notion about hypertension, including some long held by physicians, is wrong.

SYMPTOMS—AND THE LACK OF THEM

Symptoms serve a useful purpose. Hit your finger acci-
dentally with a hammer and you're in pain. Eat contam-
inated food and you're distressed. Get emotionally worked
up, tense and anxious, and you're rewarded with a headache. In each case, you're on notice that something is wrong.

Symptoms are often early-warning signals which, if unpleasant, can nevertheless be protective.

Unfortunately, whereas the body's early warning system
works for a whole host of internal and external dangers, it
falls down badly when it comes to hypertension.

Most people who know they have elevated blood pressure
know it only because it was discovered at the time of a life
insurance or other special examination, or in the course of a
routine periodic health checkup. They don't know it from
any body warnings.

Hypertension is insidious, stealthy. It may produce no
symptoms of any kind for many years. When it does produce symptoms, they may not be recognized for what they
are because they are common to many other disorders.

Headaches, including the early-morning and the back-
of-the-head types, often thought to be hypertensive in
origin, may or may not be related to blood pressure. When
they are, they do not necessarily mean that pressure is high.
In fact, in some cases, it may be very low. Many so-called
hypertensive headaches in reality stem from nervous tension; they have nothing to do with blood pressure.

Dizziness and light-headedness may be due to hypertension but they have many other possible causes. In the
same category is vertigo, which is not quite the same as
dizziness. In dizziness, there is a feeling of movement within
the head; in vertigo, the sensation is that the outside world
is moving, whirling about.

Feelings of fullness in the head, tightness over the scalp,

numbness and tingling in arms and fingers—these are also commonly thought to be indications of elevated blood pressure and may be, but not inevitably. Many a case of numbness and tingling, for example, has been cured by correcting a vitamin deficiency.

Heart palpitations, to many, mean elevated blood pressure but seldom is hypertension the cause. Nor is it a fact that people who are quick-tempered and whose veins become distended with anger are necessarily hypertensives. Anger can elevate pressure but not permanently.

Symptoms simply cannot be relied upon as early warners of hypertension.

It is true that when hypertension is well advanced, when it has been present and doing its dirty work for many years, it may finally produce severe headaches, insomnia, dizziness, vertigo, shortness of breath, and still other disturbances. When it has pounded away long enough at the delicate blood vessels in the eyes, you may experience visual disturbances, and, in fact, the degree of damage to the blood vessels of the eyes is often used by physicians as a measure of how long hypertension has been present.

Once symptoms develop, they are often symptoms of the complications of hypertension, of damage done. Treatment, then, can be helpful; it can greatly reduce mortality. But the results can't be as good as when treatment is started much earlier. Treatment can control blood pressure but it can't undo any permanent physical damage.

The damage is especially tragic when it produces severe vision impairment, or when it occurs in vital arteries, heart, or brain.

The National Heart and Lung Institute is one of the agencies currently mounting a special hypertension detection program, part of a major effort to bring to the community the fruits of years of research on high blood pressure. Dr. Theodore Cooper, its director, warns: "One's blood pressure may exist at abnormally high levels for many years without altering one's sense of health until there is serious damage, typically a stroke or heart attack, years later."

It was not untypical, for example, according to the Ameri-

can Heart Association, that during a special screening program at a large factory in Michigan, of 919 employees who
were found to have high blood pressure, 720 did not know
they had it.

WHO GETS IT?

The Young and the Old

Statistics show that hypertension is hardly a disease of
only the aged.

When, for example, Tulane University-trained students
went out into the streets of New Orleans, rang thousands of
doorbells, and took 11,309 blood pressures, they turned up
3,678 previously undiagnosed hypertensives\

Older people only?

The New Orleans survey showed a 54 percent incidence of
hypertension for people over the age of 50. But it also
showed 6 percent were 20 to 29, 16 percent were 30 to 39,
and 35 percent were 40 to 49.

Rarely, in fact, does hypertension *start* after the age of 50,
according to investigators who made a point of emphasizing that at a recent national conference on cardiovascular
diseases. The bulk of patients develop first indications of
hypertension at an average age of 30, and if it goes un-
checked, they may die of its complications at an average age
of 50 to 55.

It has been supposed, even by many physicians, that blood
pressure "inevitably" tends to go up with age and that is normal. But it is now apparent that it is not inevitable at all and
can hardly be considered normal.

For 30 years, a team of University of Alabama Medical
School investigators led by Dr. William R. Harlan, in cooperation with physicians of the U.S. Naval Aerospace Medical Research Institute, has been following up 1,056 men.
They are men who qualified for naval flight training in 1940.
All were 24 years old then. All have been examined periodically for 30 years since.

Half the men have had no blood pressure rise from ages 24 to 54. That belies the inevitability concept. Significantly, too, the study shows that when blood pressure does rise with age, it most frequently does so in those whose pressures were somewhat elevated—on the high side of what has been considered the "normal" range—to begin with.

In Chicago, investigators have been carrying out another long-term study covering men in the labor force of the People's Gas Light & Coke Co. Here, again, it has become obvious that pressure does not have to rise with age; more than 30 percent of the 900 men in the study have had no appreciable rise in 20 years. Here, again, slight elevation of pressure in youth has been shown to increase the likelihood (by as much as fivefold) that pressure will increase with age to the point of marked hypertension. And the Chicago study clearly indicates that when pressure stays steady, there is greatly reduced risk of developing heart, blood vessel, and kidney disease.

Thus, when blood pressure goes up with age, it is not normal. It is most likely to go up and reach jeopardizing levels in those in whom the level in youth was a bit high, a warning-bit high. If the warning is heeded, it does not have to advance with the years. Something can be done about it, and it is healthy to do something about it.

Adolescents and Children

When it is looked for, hypertension can be found in a surprising number of adolescents and children.

Of 435 teen-agers examined in Evans County, Georgia, 11 percent had high blood pressure. When, after seven years, investigators were able to trace 30 of those who had been found to be hypertensive and who had not had treatment, two already had died of strokes; one had hypertensive heart disease; three had developed brain and heart symptoms; five others were as yet without symptoms but had markedly elevated pressures.

Not every mild elevation in a young person necessarily means sustained hypertension. Some elevations are only temporary. But knowledgeable physicians now are convinced that there must be concern about all elevations, that they must be followed carefully, because it is impossible to predict which will be temporary and which sustained.

Hypertension has been detected in four-year-old children. Studying 40 such children, investigators at Washington University School of Medicine, St. Louis, found indications that overweight and genetic predisposition may be factors in early hypertension development. Thirty-two of the 40 children were overweight as compared to only 6 overweights in another group of 40 children with normal blood pressures. Also, in 14 of the hypertensives at least one parent was found to have elevated pressure; by contrast, only 5 in the group of normal children had a mother or father with a history of hypertension.

The Inheritors

High blood pressure is about twice as common among the brothers and sisters of hypertensives and in the children of hypertensive parents as among the relatives of people with normal pressure.

In many cases, parents or grandparents who may not have been diagnosed as having hypertension suffered from stroke or heart disease or kidney disease—any of which, it is now clear, can be a manifestation of elevated blood pressure.

Given such a family history, the chances that an individual will develop hypertension are increased, and, in fact, it is now clear that if you look for hypertension in members of such families, you may discover it at a very early age.

In 1971, Dr. Edward Kass of Harvard Medical School reported that a tendency toward hypertension can be detected as early as the age of two years in children of hypertensive parents. Kass and his colleagues measured blood pressures in 83 families with 240 children aged 2 to 14 years. The children of hypertensive parents, even at the age of 2, had higher-than-usual readings.

But not all children in a family with hypertensive history

will suffer from the disease. And many people who have no family background of hypertension develop the disease.

To cast some light on familial influences, investigators have resorted to animal studies. At Brookhaven National Laboratory, for example, Dr. Lewis K. Dahl has been able to breed one strain of rat that, under certain conditions, quickly develops hypertension, and another strain that, under the same conditions, does not develop it so readily.

Dahl's studies suggest that some of us inherit a susceptibility that can be triggered by such factors as kidney infection, emotional stress, or too much salt in the diet. Dahl says: "Where there is a family history of hypertension, it behooves a person to avoid the possible precipitating factors by limiting salt intake, carefully treating kidney infections, and minimizing emotional stress. This last can be difficult, I know—domineering bosses and quarrelsome mothers-in-law may be hard to avoid."

Actually, although the evidence is strong that inherited susceptibility may play a role when there is a family pattern of hypertension, the influence of family environment has to be considered. If there is inheritance, it is not of elevated blood pressure itself but of one or more of the many mechanisms that may influence the blood pressure level. But families eat together, live together, and their members interact with each other. And even without an inherited susceptibility, it is possible that family-shared eating patterns, living habits, etc., may account for a higher incidence of hypertension in some families than in others.

Male and Female

Hypertension does not belong to either sex exclusively, although there is an impression shared by many people that it is far more common among women.

But a national health survey by the Public Health Service does not bear this out.

Indeed, at the ages of 18 to 24, 10.9 percent of the men versus 1.4 percent of the women have hypertension; at ages *scale closer as all?*

25 to 34, the incidence is 11.9 percent for men, 3.2 percent for women; at ages 35 to 44, 14.2 percent for men, 9 percent for women; from 45 to 54, 17.7 percent for men and 15.3 percent for women; from 55 to 64, 27.5 percent for men and 24.5 percent for women; from 65 to 74, 24.8 percent for men, 24.3 percent for women. Finally, in the age range 75 to 79, women outdo men, with 28.3 percent incidence versus the male 26.7 percent.

Women and the Pill

In some young women, it now appears that hypertension may develop as a complication of using oral contraceptives. Doctors have been reporting finding significant hypertension in some, but not by any means all, women using the Pill. The blood pressure may rise weeks to months after start of use; usually it falls by four weeks after the Pill has been discontinued.

How often the complication occurs is not known. One study found a significant rise in pressure in about 20 percent of women using oral contraceptives. Whether or not that is typical, the study does focus attention on the need to measure, at least occasionally, the blood pressure of every woman using the Pill, an editorial in the *Journal of the American Medical Association* points out.

Black and White

2nd par

While hypertension occurs in both blacks and whites, for unknown reasons it is not only more frequent among black people but also, for them, develops earlier in life, is often more severe, and causes higher mortality at younger ages.

In the District of Columbia, for example 65 percent of the population is black, but 75 percent of the 645 deaths in one year attributed to hypertension occurred among blacks. Of the deaths due to hypertension, 239 occurred in persons under 60 and 88 percent of these were blacks.

Dr. Frank A. Finnerty, who heads Georgetown University's Cardiovascular Group at the District of Columbia

General Hospital, headed a team that examined 289 young black women (average age, 23 years) selected at random from patients attending the hospital's birth control clinic. One hundred forty-one, 48 percent, had hypertension. "This finding," says Dr. Finnerty, "is shockingly high and has great socioeconomic importance. It is these young women who will have strokes at an early age if their conditions go unnoticed and untreated."

More or Less Active Men?

To find out, Dr. Henry J. Montoye, of the University of Michigan, studied 1,696 men, aged 20 to 64. After being interviewed intensively about their work and leisure activities, the men were classified according to degree of activity.

Blood pressures were significantly lower in active men than in sedentary. But men who worked 40 hours or less each week had lower pressures than those who worked 40 to 50 hours, and men who worked more than 50 hours a week had the highest pressures.

A Distinctive Personality Type for Hypertension?

Some investigators believe so. Most prone to hypertension, they indicate, may be the individual who experiences emotional upsets more often, more intensively, and for longer periods than other people do.

At the University of California, San Francisco, a group of college women who had undergone physicals during registration were found to have hypertension. They were carefully interviewed at that point, four years later, and again 11 years later.

The interviews established four apparently significant characteristics in the hypertensive women. They have a "low threshold" for perceiving hostility in others, for retaliating, and for behaving in ways likely to provoke anger in other people. They have a hidden but unremitting kind of anxious, tense, defensive attitude. They fail to achieve roles appropriate for their age and sex. And they tend to overrespond to many types of stimuli such as irritability, anxiety, and restlessness. And the higher the women scored in the four categories, the higher were their blood pressures.

In a study with U.S. Air Force officers, those with highest blood pressures were "dominant, assertive, decisive, task-oriented, and generally tended to be effective in their leadership roles." But when they were matched with other officers with similar leadership qualities but lower blood pressures, the higher-pressure men, by comparison, "tended to have narrow ranges of interest, low thresholds for perceiving threat, challenge and hostility in other people, and were overcontrolling, rigid, stereotyped, and obtuse in their social relationships." As did the college women, the officers with higher blood pressures had high levels of emotional arousal.

Though there is no doubt that emotional stimuli can cause blood pressure to rise in both normal people and hypertensives, generally the increases in hypertensives are believed to be greater than in the normotensives.

Yet, whereas many investigators favor the idea that hypertensives tend to be people whose emotions are stronger and their greater pressure elevations result from the larger amounts of emotion they generate, others think that what may be involved is a greater reactivity, or sensitivity, of the heart and blood vessel system in hypertensives so that a given emotional stimuli may produce a greater increase in pressure.

It may well be that both explanations are correct for different individuals.

WHEN IS BLOOD PRESSURE TOO HIGH?
OLD CUTOFF POINTS AND NEW VIEWS

How high *is* high blood pressure? How far up does the pressure have to go to signal danger?

There is a whole new picture now, markedly different from what it was only a few years ago. It is now being recognized that the old cutoff points between the normal and safe on the one hand and the abnormal and unsafe on the other hand were unrealistic.

It is also being recognized by some investigators that it may not be one pressure, the diastolic, the pressure between heartbeats, the lower pressure you see written in a blood pressure report, for example, the 90 in 140/90, that alone is critical, as long believed. The systolic pressure, the pressure when the heart beats, the higher pressure noted in blood pressure reports, may also be of importance.

Whereas the 1959 Society of Actuaries study of the lives and deaths of almost 4 million life insurance policyholders was a landmark in the developing story of hypertension and its significance, it came at a time when some of its indications had to be tempered because of practical realities.

The study clearly established the high incidence of elevated blood pressure even among the middle-aged and young; it established the great influence of hypertension on life expectancy. It also produced evidence that even very mildly increased blood pressure levels could have significant effects, for example, that men 35 years of age with blood pressure of 142/85 tended to have a death rate about 150 percent above average for their age.

The study came at a time when modern drugs to treat elevated pressure were just beginning to appear. Only a few years before, there was little in the way of effective medication. Surgery had been used in very severe cases of hypertension, but it was no light matter and was not advocated for milder elevations. By 1959 there were a few useful drugs, but they were potent, could produce undesirable effects in some patients, and they, too, were reserved for what were considered significant blood pressure elevations.

In this atmosphere, although the Society of Actuaries study suggested that 140/90 might mark the upper limit of normal pressure, it seemed practical to accept that but also to establish a kind of borderline area between 140/90 and 160/95, and to consider that there should be real concern and active treatment for pressure above 160/95. In fact, this was the definition of hypertension established by the World Health Organization: 160/95 and higher.

But then came the more recent studies that have helped to change medical thinking about hypertension, including how high pressure has to be to be potentially dangerous and to warrant close attention.

THE NEW FINDINGS

The Framingham study has been referred to several times already. It is a study of major importance, large in scope, long in term, and the data from it are continuously being analyzed and re-analyzed.

For example, in the first 14 years of the study, out of the thousands examined, 65 of the men and 70 of the women experienced strokes, and first analysis revealed that the stroke risk was about five times as high among those with blood pressure levels greater than 160/95 than among those with levels under 140/90.

But then, as the data were analyzed still further, it became evident that there was no neat cutoff point, no one critical level beyond which blood pressure suddenly became dangerous. The risk was simply proportional to the pressure level even within the borderline area below 160/95.

The second phase of the 17-hospital Veterans Administration study headed by Dr. Freis has also provided some evidence of the importance of mild pressure elevations. After the first phase had shown a marked reduction in stroke, congestive heart failure, and other serious or deadly events among treated men with diastolic blood pressures above 115, the second phase showed a dramatic reduction in such events among treated men with diastolic pressures in the 90 through 114 range.

When the VA analysis was completed, it indicated that for patients with diastolic pressures even only a few points above 90, the risk of developing a major heart or blood vessel complication over a 5-year period was reduced two-thirds by treatment.

According to these and other studies, it now appears that a person with mild hypertension has twice the normal risk of dying before he is 65—which, as mentioned earlier, translates (according to Dr. Edward Frohlich of the University of Oklahoma) into a decrease of up to 17 years in the life expectancy of a 35-year-old man.

Emphasizing the importance of mild elevations, Dr. William B. Kannel, director of the Framingham study, declares: "All cutoffs are artificial. The risk is on a continuous gradient, proportional to the blood pressure level. An ideal blood pressure would be the lowest pressure you could achieve without going into shock."

And, in all seriousness, Dr. Kannel adds: "People with low blood pressure may complain that they're tired all the time, but they live for 120 years."

There is still some debate among physicians about the blood pressure level at which active treatment should begin. Late in 1971, however, a respected study group, part of the Intersociety Commission on Heart Disease Resources, chose 140 or greater systolic or 90 or greater diastolic pressure as the point at which to do further tests of a patient and, if not treated, to keep the patient under protective close watch.

HEEDING THAT UPPER—
SYSTOLIC—PRESSURE

It has long been assumed by medical people, with seemingly good reason, that diastolic pressure is the significant measurement and the systolic pressure is of much lesser importance.

Though the systolic is the higher pressure, occurring with the heartbeat at the moment when blood is ejected from the heart into the arteries, the diastolic, or between-beat, pressure is still the one to which the arteries are subjected for the longest periods. Therefore, it would seem that the diastolic, if elevated, might produce the major share of damage.

Also, it has been long believed that systolic pressure tends to go up naturally with age—recall the common belief that when systolic pressure equals the sum of 100 and a person's age, it is a normal systolic pressure.

But a 60-year-old with 160 systolic no longer can be considered to have a normal pressure, nor can a 45-year-old with 145.

A systolic pressure does *not* necessarily increase normally with age, and any systolic pressure above 140 at *any* age has to be viewed with some concern.

And there is new evidence that the systolic pressure is important. In the Framingham study, it proved to be as important as the diastolic.

With thorough analysis of the Framingham data, it turned out that there were similar degrees of risk for coronary heart disease regardless of whether people were classified by their systolic or diastolic pressures. Neither systolic and diastolic pressures combined nor any other pressure determinations and combinations proved to be any more accurate in predicting risk than systolic measurements alone. In fact, the relative significance of diastolic pressure in terms of coronary heart disease risk, the Framingham study suggests, actually may tend to decline with age while the significance of the systolic pressure may increase.

Recently, Framingham researchers have urged the reevaluation of the current practice of assessing the importance of blood pressure at all ages largely on the basis of the diastolic measurement; also of regarding elevated systolic pressure as innocuous in the elderly.

GETTING AT THE PROBLEM

What makes hypertension so much of a problem and challenge bears reemphasizing. It is not that it is dangerous and common—it is more common than previously believed and potentially dangerous at levels below those once thought to be the hazard levels. Neglect is the problem. In the vast majority of cases, from mildest to most severe, hypertension is a controllable disorder, often readily controllable, and in some cases even curable, as the next several chapters show.

5

Kinds and Causes

One of the most dramatic advances of modern medicine—dramatic from the standpoint of snatching patients from the jaws of death—is the control of one kind of hypertension that used to kill its victims very quickly.

Malignant hypertension, as it is called, is relatively rare. The likelihood that any reader of this book will have it is small. Yet the advance against malignant hypertension illustrates something important about most of hypertension.

Malignant hypertension knows no age boundaries but occurs more often in the young than in the old. The pressure is usually very high. Vision is affected; there may be fits and paroxysms of breathlessness. Kidney function declines rapidly. Once it was a matter of months, or a year or so at best, between the time malignant hypertension was diagnosed and death.

No longer. Most patients with malignant hypertension today can look forward to useful lives. Yet there are great gaps in the understanding of why malignant hypertension develops, what causes it.

It would be nice if those gaps could be closed. Undoubtedly, they will be. Meanwhile, for practical purposes, for lifesaving, no matter the gaps, control is what counts, and control can be achieved now.

All other hypertension is distinguished from the malignant by the term "benign." It is not the best of terms. Nonmalignant hypertension moves slowly; the pressure is not as high as in malignant; there may be no symptoms at all for many years—no vision disturbances, no fits, no paroxysms

61

of breathlessness, no other obvious indications of any kind. Nevertheless, nonmalignant hypertension, as we have already seen, can be producing its complications, playing its significant role in clogging arteries, paving the way for stroke, heart attack, congestive heart failure, kidney failure, and the rest. It is NOT benign.

But the term sticks, and actually, it is a catchall term.

There is more than one kind of benign hypertension, from the standpoint of causes, known and unknown. In benign hypertension, as in malignant, even though there are still great gaps in knowledge about causes, effective control is possible.

While research scientists work constantly to get a better grip on understanding what brings on elevations of pressure, the elevations have become controllable so that the complications of the elevations become controllable. And such control of benign hypertension promises to be no less dramatically valuable from a lifesaving standpoint in the long run than the control of malignant.

As an analogy, a constant headache or backache can wreak havoc in a person's life. It can interfere with his sleep, work, family and social life, and make him emotionally upset. These are its complications. If the cause of the headache or backache can be pinpointed and then eliminated, that's the most desirable. If it can't, and until it can be, then clearly the next best thing is to relieve the ache and avoid the complications.

And so it is today with most cases of hypertension.

SOME KNOWN CAUSES

In the overwhelming majority of people with hypertension, as many as 90 percent or even more of them, no physical cause can be found as yet.

We've seen that if, for any reason, the tiny arterioles clamp tight in wholesale fashion all over the body, blood pressure goes up and stays up, and the result is hypertension.

But in only a small percentage of cases can the hypertension be traced to a specific disease.

In some cases, a kidney infection may lead to elevation of blood pressure. Obstruction of an artery feeding a kidney may do the same. Atop the kidneys are the small but vital adrenal glands, and disorders of the adrenals can cause hypertension. Another uncommon cause is constriction (coarctation) of the aorta, the great artery emerging from the heart.

As mentioned earlier, when such definite physical causes of hypertension can be found, the hypertension often can be cured once and for all by medical or surgical treatment of the causes. We will pay more detailed attention to these causes, how they are diagnosed, and the treatments for them in the next chapter.

Here we are concerned with by far the most common kind of hypertension, which does not seem to have any connection with any other disease. It is called "essential" hypertension. But the word "essential" is used not in the ordinary sense of being indispensable, something absolutely needed, but rather in the medical sense of being independent of a local cause. Another medical term for such hypertension is "idiopathic," which means a primary disease without apparent cause.

There must, of course, be factors involved in producing essential hypertension. And though researchers have no final answers yet, they are following many leads.

A MATTER OF HEREDITY? FURTHER INSIGHTS

There seems little doubt that heredity is involved in hypertension but the extent to which it is and the mode or modes of inheritance are still not entirely clear.

Some investigators have looked upon heredity as possibly a main cause. They have considered hypertension to be a disorder, basically, of middle age, reflecting the operation of a single gene, the unit of heredity transmission.

According to their view, some people do not inherit the particular gene for hypertension from either parent and in such persons blood pressure rises little if at all with increasing years. Some inherit the gene from one parent and develop a moderate pressure elevation. Those who inherit the gene from both parents develop severe hypertension.

Other investigators believe that blood pressure is determined by many genetic and environmental factors, all more or less equal in importance.

Though it is unquestionably true those persons whose parents had high blood pressure are more likely to develop it than those whose parents did not have high blood pressure, families have more in common than genes. We've already mentioned these—environmental factors, such as food and living conditions. Environmental factors may affect susceptibility to hypertension, particularly when the environmental factors interact with any hereditary predisposition.

The situation may be not entirely unlike that for body height. Whereas it is commonly seen that a tendency toward tallness or shortness runs in families, it is also true that a person's height is determined partly by his environment. For example, in increasingly affluent countries, children tend to be taller than their parents.

The influence of heredity in hypertension has been shown in many types of studies. For one thing, the blood pressures of identical twins, with exactly the same inheritance, have been found to resemble each other much more than do the blood pressures of nonidentical twins who, of course, do not share exactly the same hereditary characteristics.

Among patients diagnosed as having hypertension at a mean age of 36½ years, it turned out that 44 percent of the parents had been hypertensive. But when a group of subjects of the same age and free of hypertension were checked, only 14 percent of their parents were hypertensive.

It is possible, in such ways as feeding salt solutions or damaging a kidney or part of a kidney, to produce hypertension in normal rats. But when pressure-raising measures were applied to rats with inherited, or genetic, hypertension, bred for the purpose, they produced higher eventual blood pressures than when they were applied to the normal rats.

In the studies of first-degree relatives of hypertensive patients over a period of time, they were compared with subjects representative of the general population. The rise with age of blood pressure was significantly greater in the relatives of hypertensive patients than in the others, indicating that in man increasing pressure with age is influenced to an important degree by genetic factors as it is in rats with genetic hypertension.

But how exactly do hereditary influences work? There are still no definitive answers, but Dr. Caroline C. Bedell Thomas of Johns Hopkins Hospital has suggested that it is more plausible to think of hereditary predisposition to hypertension not as a matter of some one gene but rather of a number of genes interacting. Genes concerned with nervous system, glands, blood vessels, kidneys, may interact in different combinations and degrees, giving rise to a predisposition toward hypertension.

IS IT A MATTER OF SALT AND HEREDITY?

For more than 20 years, some investigators, notably Dr. Lewis K. Dahl, who bred the colonies of hypertensive rats, have been working on the concept that chronic excess intake of salt may cause hypertension. And recently they have reported studies indicating that genetic factors may determine who will and who will not tolerate a high salt intake.

"By the chronic eating of salt," says Dahl, "we're talking about what most people call table salt. Chemically, it's sodium chloride, and this may be added at the table or it may be added in the kitchen by the cook, it may be added by the processor of foods—in other words, it can be added anywhere along the line after nature gets done with it. It's of interest that natural foods do not contain high salt, so that you can only consume a high salt diet if somewhere along the line man has added it to the food."

Dahl first became interested in salt in 1948 when a rice-fruit diet was being used with some good results to treat hypertension. What was the ingredient in the diet that accounted for the pressure-lowering effect? In four years of studies, Dahl and other investigators discovered that it was not some special ingredient *in* the diet but rather its very low salt content. Studies showed that when the same diet was used but with salt added, there was no beneficial effect on hypertension.

Dahl began to wonder. If a low salt intake could produce a lowering of blood pressure, might a high salt intake be a cause of hypertension?

By 1950 there were a number of studies showing the effectiveness of salt restriction in hypertension. Most agreed that about one-third of the patients had an excellent response, one-third only a modest response, one-third had little or no response.

Since then, over the many years in which he has seen hypertensive patients, Dahl has reported that he has never seen a new patient who was on a low salt intake.

But high salt intake is common in our society. The custom of adding salt to food is ancient. The appetite for salt, however, Dahl points out, is acquired and the appetite adapts itself to individual salt intake. Among his patients, Dahl reports, have been some who felt compelled to add salt to their food "until it looked like snow" and one patient confessed that he salted bacon and potato chips just to make sure!

There have been some who have argued that since animals sometimes make long treks to salt licks, there is an inborn salt appetite that must have continued in man. But only herbivores, Dahl notes, make such treks. "The omnivores and carnivores may go to licks, too, not in search of salt but in search of herbivores! The salt hunger of the herbivores, furthermore, is often due to true salt deficiency; with a few exceptions, all plants are low in sodium. In areas far removed from the sea, the soil can become leached of salt. The plants will, therefore, have extremely low sodium contents."

Dahl is convinced that salt appetites are acquired and

that the high salt intakes now so common do not reflect body needs.

Because of the large amount of salt almost uniformly consumed in the United States from childhood to old age, it is difficult to establish clearly how much of a role salt intake plays in causing hypertension in a given individual because the factor is common to all. In man, Dahl acknowledges, it is possible to state only that there is a relationship between salt intake and elevated pressure, but in the rat, the cause and effect relationship is clearly demonstrable.

Over the past 20 years, Dahl has worked with more than 32,000 rats. Thousands developed hypertension from chronic salt feeding. As the work went on, Dahl noticed that in unselected rats the response to salt ranged all the way from no effect at all to gradually increasing pressures to rapidly malignant hypertension. About one-quarter of the animals showed no elevation of pressure even after consuming a very high salt diet most of their lives. The remaining three-quarters developed elevations of varying degrees, including 2 to 3 percent dying of hypertension after just a few months on salt.

This suggested genetic variances—hereditary influences. So Dahl and his colleagues started mating members at either extreme of the response range and within a few generations had two colonies, which they have since kept breeding and studying.

In one colony, the rats—called R, or resistant, strain—generally show a lack of response to high salt intake; the average blood pressure of the group is not significantly increased. In the other colony—the S, or sensitive strain—moderate amounts of salt in the diet produce significant rises in blood pressure and high salt intake leads to death in a few months.

Such experiments indicate that heredity can be a critical factor in determining whether or not experimental hypertension develops. Certainly, in rats, when heredity is suitable and some appropriate nonhereditary factor such as high salt intake is present, hypertension is more likely to develop than if there were hereditary resistance.

If this applies to man, as it clearly does in rats, Dr. Dahl suggests, at one extreme there should be people with so strong a genetic predisposition as to need only very little in the way of environmental stimuli such as salt intake to develop hypertension and at the other extreme there should be people with such weak predisposition by heredity that they might fail to develop hypertension even after intense and prolonged exposure to environmental stimuli so bad for others. But most people will fall in between. The usual person will be one with only a modest predisposition who may or may not develop hypertension depending upon such things as the severity and duration of the inciting factors, such as salt intake.

IS IT A MATTER OF WATER?

Can the hardness or softness of water have anything to do with hypertension?

It may.

Attention was first directed to water in 1957 when a Japanese scientist observed that areas in Japan where the river water was more acid had a higher incidence of stroke than areas where the water was less acid.

After this observation, a follow-up in the United States showed that states served by soft water had higher death rates from heart and blood vessel diseases than states served by hard water. Other studies showed the same relationship in England, Finland, Canada, Sweden, and, to a lesser extent, in the Netherlands and Ireland.

If such a relationship were found in only one country, it might have been a fortuitous statistical association not related to cause and effect. Since it was found in several countries, it could be more than a chance matter. Something in the water, or associated with it, may influence heart and blood vessel function. In terms of hypertension in particular, some U.S. findings indicate that the harder the water, the lower the death rate from hypertensive heart disease.

If soft water is a culprit, why? It may be a matter of a

trace metal, suggests Dr. Henry Schroeder of Dartmouth Medical School who has long been interested in the influence of various such metals on health and disease.

Trace metals are those which appear in water and foods in minute quantities. Some are vital. For example, only a minute amount of copper, on the order of just 1/10 of a gram, 3/1000s of an ounce, stands between us and death because copper is essential for blood formation. Just one part of fluoride per million parts of drinking water is beneficial for dental health, offering some protection against decay. Recently, trace amounts of zinc have been found to speed the healing of wounds.

Water hardness is determined by its calcium and magnesium content and increases as the quantities of the two metals increase. But Dr. Schroeder blames soft water not for its lack of the two metals but because it has a high content of another trace metal, cadmium. Whereas hard water lays down a protective lime coating in water pipes, soft water does not but instead picks up some carbon dioxide in the air, becomes slightly acid and, because of the slight acidity, dissolves cadmium from pipes. And people with hypertension have been found to have higher concentrations of cadmium in their kidneys than people with normal blood pressure.

An alternative explanation for any influence soft water may have on the development of hypertension is that it may not contain various beneficial minerals present in hard water.

Some experts note that before getting too excited about any "water factor," a word of caution is in order. The World Health Organization's Cardiovascular Disease Unit has recently pointed out that the amount of water we drink as such, under usual conditions in affluent societies, is rather limited. Much of our fluid intake comes from various other drinks such as milk, wine, beer, soft beverages, fruit juices, coffee, and tea, and also from water contained in vegetables, fruits, and other foods. Much water is used for cooking and minerals may be deposited on, or extracted from, food being cooked. In all these drinks and foods, mineral amounts may be quite different from what they are in tap water and they are more important sources of minerals than the water we drink.

Moreover, the World Health Organization unit points out another problem. The primary source of all minerals is rocks. The mineral composition of rocks influences, through complex relationships, the chemical composition not only of water but also of the top soil layer and, eventually, the mineral composition of plants growing in these soils and of animals feeding on these plants. A mineral deficiency or abundance in the geological environment could possibly produce a deficiency or abnormal uptake of certain minerals by man. This is still only a tentative theory, but some evidence of the ill effect of certain geochemical environments on human health has been found. The incidence of several diseases has been reported to be associated with the occurrence of certain rock types deficient in one or another element. Preliminary studies in the United States suggest that death rates from heart and blood vessel diseases are higher in areas where soils are generally poor in trace elements, lower in areas underlain by certain rocks which, through weathering, continuously contribute a good supply of trace elements to the soil.

And other preliminary findings indicate that several countries with high heart and blood vessel disease rates are underlain by rocks of older geologic age, and older rocks tend to produce soft water because they consist largely of relatively insoluble minerals, such as lead, and the soil that covers them may contain few minerals.

"All these bits and pieces of evidence," the WHO unit notes, "point to a relationship between the chemical composition of the environment (be it rocks, soil, water, or food) and cardiovascular diseases through trace element imbalance . . . These are all-important problems. They deserve deeper investigations on a multi-disciplinary, international scale, and WHO is already carrying out work in this direction."

If and when such investigations provide enough firm facts, they could open the way to changing trace element environment and dietary habits. Fluoridation of water, addition of iodine to table salt, and addition of vitamins to certain foods are examples of such changes already made.

But the WHO unit, like other authoritative medical sources, considers that it is still premature to advocate such actions in the field of hypertension and heart and blood vessel diseases in general.

IS IT A MATTER OF OBESITY?

Physicians have long had the impression that hypertension and obesity—a common problem in the United States and in virtually all affluent countries—may be related.

The Framingham, Massachusetts, study has confirmed this impression.

Framingham people with hypertension were found to be more obese than people with normal blood pressure. Also, the prevalence of hypertension at all ages increased with relative weight. It made no difference what measure of excessive fat, or adiposity, was used—relative weight, skin fold, or upper arm girth: the average blood pressure level increased with the degree of excessive fat.

The Framingham study showed that risk of hypertension was distinctly related to weight gain. It also showed that the relationship between obesity and hypertension is complex. Not only did obese subjects develop an excess of hypertension but lean hypertensive patients had an increased tendency to get fat. This suggests that both obesity and hypertension may be related to some third factor. Significantly, however, from both a prevention and treatment standpoint, people who lost weight had a fall in blood pressure. About 60 percent of hypertensives who were able to achieve a substantial weight loss were able to lose their hypertensive blood pressure levels.

As noted earlier, in Chapter 4, investigators working with children with hypertension have found that excess weight is a factor in the development of elevated pressure levels.

Similarly, in the 30-year study of men who qualified for naval flight training in 1940 carried out by Dr. William R.

Harlan of the University of Alabama Medical School and
other investigators (see also Chapter 4), weight has stood
out as a major factor in those who became hypertensive.
The greatest increase in weight occurred between the ages
of 24 and 36, and blood pressure increases were greatest during this period. Moreover, the relationship of weight gain to
blood pressure was found to remain significant throughout
adult life.

WHAT OF RACE?

In addition to the study in Washington, D.C., showing
that hypertension occurs, for unknown reasons, more often
in blacks than whites, and at earlier ages and in more severe
forms (see Chapter 4), other studies have shown a national
prevalence of hypertension among blacks twice as high as in
the white population.

One particularly searching study has been done in Charleston, S.C., where, according to the 1960 census, 36 percent of
the population consists of Gullah Negroes who appear to be
closer to West African Negroes than the average American
Negro. Charleston Negroes have had markedly higher death
rates from hypertensive disease than American Negroes in
general and rates 10 to 20 times those of the total U.S.
population.

Recently investigators marked out a representative sample of 2,500 persons, blacks and whites, in the Charleston
area. They used a 23-foot trailer to perform complete examinations near the residences of subjects, thus encouraging cooperation.

They found considerable differences between the whites
and blacks. With white men and women, diastolic blood
pressure tended to ascend gradually with age. Among the
blacks, systolic pressure was significantly greater than for
the whites. The pressures of black women were significantly
higher than those for black men and increased more sharply
with age. Diastolic pressure in the blacks showed a notable

increase with age in the earlier years, prior to any appreciable rise in whites.

In whites, there is a gradual rise in the prevalence of definite diastolic hypertension with increasing body weight; the rate of rise is comparable for both men and women. But in blacks there is no such clear correlation between body weight and hypertension. Moreover, there is a marked disparity in the pressure-weight relationship of black men compared with black women. This is particularly pronounced among the underweight and the prevalence of hypertension in underweight black women is five times that for men.

The study showed that at the ages of 35 to 44, Charleston black men had 10 times the white incidence of diastolic pressures greater than 100; in men aged 65 years or more, about 6 times as many blacks had such pressures. Among women aged 35 to 44, 4 times as many blacks had such elevations as did whites; at ages 65 or more, 37 percent of black as against 11 percent of white women had such elevations.

An instrument that estimates the degree of skin pigmentation, a photoelectric reflectance colorimeter, was used, indicating slightly lighter skin for black women than men—a difference that could be occupational or hormonal in nature. A significantly greater prevalence of above-normal pressures was found in the darker half of the black population. In the 45-to-54 age bracket, more than 70 percent of darker men had above-normal pressures. A similar prevalence among lighter men was not reached until 10 years later.

Yet some studies de-emphasize any genetic or racial factor as the explanation for why blacks are more prone to hypertension.

One study by University of Michigan investigators covers carefully selected Detroit residents, some 1,524 of them, chosen from four different neighborhoods: a white high-stress area, a black high-stress area, a middle-class-white low-stress area, and a middle-class-black low-stress area. Stress was rated on the basis of crime rates, income, education, employment rates, divorce and separation rates, density of population, and mobility.

Eventually, the hope is that results of the study, after thorough analysis, may give some indication of how much hypertension is due to genetics and how much to the environment. But already there are indications that black men and women in relatively good Detroit neighborhoods have a significantly lower incidence of hypertension than do those in high-stress neighborhoods.

STRESS AND HYPERTENSION

During a great oil fire in Texas, a major earthquake in Iran, and the siege of Leningrad by the Germans in World War II, the incidence of hypertension was found to have increased as much as 300 percent.

The increase is no surprise. That stressful situations and strong emotions can cause blood pressure elevations has been well documented.

For example, using equipment that could continuously monitor blood pressure, investigators studied the reactions of a pilot who was about to make a test flight when at the last minute his plane developed some mechanical trouble. For four hours, the pilot waited while technicians tried to find what was wrong. In that time, increasingly, as he became more and more impatient and frustrated, his blood pressure rose. Once the plane was repaired and he could get on with his job, his blood pressure dropped.

Another pilot, also monitored for blood pressure in the same way, showed a 50 percent rise immediately after he overheard a remark, deliberately made, which he took to be disparaging.

Researchers have also registered the blood pressures of several dozen men whose jobs were threatened. They took pressure measurements for each man not only during the time he was expecting to lose his job but also when he had lost it, during the time he was out of work, during trial re-employment, and finally when he had a regular job again. They found that the men's pressures stayed elevated all through the time of stress—from the time of threatened job loss right through to the time when they were back at regular work. Only when they felt secure once more, did pressure drop. It was notable, too, that the expectation of losing a job produced as great an increase in pressure as did the actual losing of a job.

Among the healthiest, longest-lived people on earth, despite the fact that they get little medical care, are the Mabaans, a tribe living in the Sudan. Does their way of life—isolated from outside influences, apparently happily adapted to their environment, with little of the stress known to Western culture—spare them many illnesses? So believe investigators who report that the Mabaans, including many of the oldest among them, have virtually perfect vision and hearing, and blood pressures that remain normal, unchanged, throughout life.

Investigators who have studied hypertension for years and believe it to be closely related to stressful emotional disturbances report such cases as that of a young woman who had determined that her marriage would not be like her parents', full of quarreling and bitterness. But she married a man who turned out to be a rigid and critical husband. To keep peace she had to defer to him in everything. She nursed her baby and nursed her grievances; she tried losing herself in community activities, and, despite her unhappiness and her husband's behavior, appeared to be relaxed and affable. But she developed dangerously high blood pressure. Finally, she exploded, released all her pent-up resentment against her husband, divorced him, and subsequently remarried. Her blood pressure returned to normal.

Some years ago, in experiments at Michael Reese Hospital, Chicago, persons with normal blood pressure were deliberately exposed to anger-producing situations. In those who bottled up their anger, blood pressure shot up; in those who freely expressed anger, there was much less elevation.

In a wide variety of laboratory episodes of emotional stress, investigators have been able to document the effects on blood pressure. They have found, for example, that in a group of hypertensive women, interviews covering their personal histories and current life situations triggered increases of as much as 40 points and more in pressure. Of course there were variations from woman to woman and from one moment to another in the same woman, with the latter variations being closely related to the degree to which the subject got emotionally involved with the interviewer and with the topics under discussion.

To extend such studies to longer periods of observation and to naturally occurring life situations, investigators developed a portable type of blood pressure recorder so that subjects could make records of their pressures on a preset schedule, usually every half hour, as they went about ordinary activities outside the laboratory. The subjects also kept logs of their activities, checking a list of adjectives describing several moods or attitudes after each pressure measurement: anxiety, hostility, depression, feeling of time pressure (all negative affects), and alertness and contentment (positive affects). The blood pressures were consistently and markedly higher whenever negative affects were reported in the logs.

A group of male executives and office workers were followed for two days through their mostly sedentary workdays and into the evenings. Under emotional stress, the pressure for the average man increased by about 50 points and in some cases by more than 80.

In the past, some researchers thought that such stress-induced episodes of pressure elevation might have little relevance to the development of hypertension since the pressure changes were believed to be due simply to an increase in the heart's output of blood and did not involve constriction of blood vessels. But then came studies showing that at least in some people the pressure increase is brought about by blood vessel resistance as well as increased blood output.

Because of such findings, it seems reasonable to many scientists to believe that some people, because of personality characteristics, may be especially likely to overrespond in emotion-producing situations and, as a result, are subject to more frequent, greater, and longer-lasting elevation episodes which, over a period of time, could lead to sustained hypertension. $S + \circ P$

As the American Heart Association has pointed out: Wrapped up somehow in the whole business of high blood pressure is the subject of emotion. When a person is angry or afraid, his blood pressure may go up. It may increase just because he knows he is going to have his blood pressure taken. Rises like these, during times of stress, are perfectly normal. But some individuals react to even mild life stresses with an excessive rise in blood pressure. (When the stress has passed, the blood pressure returns to normal.) These men and women are called hyper-reactors or pre-hypertensives. Chances are that in time many of them will develop hypertension. Their bodies simply get used to responding to daily life as if it were a series of emergencies."] Foot Note

The relationship of personality to hypertension and other health problems has been considered in many studies.

Patients with seven different conditions, one of which was essential hypertension, were interviewed. The interviews were recorded and the transcripts then were carefully edited by physicians to eliminate any material having to do with physical symptoms or providing any kind of medical clue that might reveal the diagnosis.

A panel of psychiatrists then judged each interview and identified all the conditions, including hypertension, far better than would be possible by chance. Next, a group of physicians studied the same transcripts. They identified only 25 percent of the diagnoses, indicating that the removal of medical clues had indeed been successful and that the psychological information used for psychiatric interpretation permitted valid inferences about the diagnoses.

The picture of the hypertensive personality that permitted the psychiatrists to correctly identify the hypertensive patients was that of an individual continuously struggling against expressing his hostile, aggressive feelings, and having difficulty asserting himself. After an often stormy childhood with attacks of rage and aggression, the individual had developed a more submissive, compliant attitude. The overly conscientious, responsible attitude had resulted in increased resentment, demanding greater and greater control of hostile feelings. It was a vicious cycle, leading to chronic psychological tension.

At the Chicago Institute for Psychoanalysis since 1932, investigators have been studying emotional conflicts in people with various diseases. They have found, for example, that the asthma victim often fears losing a parent, that the neurodermatitis sufferer may have a great unmet craving for physical closeness, that the person prone to rheumatoid arthritis is one who has trouble handling aggressive feelings—and while trying to hold these feelings in check still manages to exercise a kind of benevolent tyranny over others and may develop the arthritis when, for any reason, a dominated person is lost. People with hypertension, the findings suggest, bottle up hostile impulses, tend to be overconscientious, to work hard and invite increasing loads, and to live in a state of tension and increasing resentment.

In their recent book, *Psychosomatics* (Viking, New York, 1972), Howard R. and Martha E. Lewis tell of the work of psychiatrist Floyd O. Ring of the University of Nebraska College of Medicine who started out with grave reservations about the validity of any supposed correlations between personality and physical ailments. It seemed to him that it was a simple matter for an investigator, armed with the knowledge that a person had some particular condition, whether hypertension or a peptic ulcer, to pick out characteristics to support a preconceived idea of a personality pattern.

So Ring had colleagues refer to him more than 400 patients suffering from a wide variety of ailments, ranging from asthma and backache to migraine, ulcer, arthritis, and hypertension. The patients were under instructions to give no information to Ring about their symptoms, disabilities, anything at all connected with their physical condition. And always, during an interview, the body of the patient was covered so there was no visible hint of physical condition.

Ring was astonished at how many correct diagnoses he

could arrive at, based on personality alone, after a 15-to-25-minute interview.

After successfully diagnosing the majority of patients, his analysis showed that personality types could be divided into three broad categories: the excessive reactors, the deficient reactors, and the restrained reactors.

For example, an individual is asked what he would do if, when he was sitting on a park bench minding his own business, a stranger walked up and without provocation kicked him in the shins. The excessive reactor wouldn't bother to ask for a reasonable explanation. Instead he would "have a showdown" or "beat hell out of him." In this category, Ring found, were all the victims of peptic ulcer, degenerative arthritis, and coronary occlusion.

When the deficient reactors were asked what they would do, their usual response was "nothing." In this group fell most of those suffering from neurodermatitis, rheumatoid arthritis, and ulcerative colitis.

The restrained reactors characteristically might respond by saying, "I'd be pretty mad" or "I might hit him." Aware of fears and angers, they rarely expressed or acted on them. In this group, Ring found, fell most sufferers from asthma, diabetes, migraine, hyperthyroidism—and hypertension.

HYPERTENSION AND
"THE GAMES PEOPLE PLAY"

"Within the family, or outside it," believes a Los Angeles physiologist, "the most powerful source of emotional disturbance is other people." And therein may lie the cause of hypertension, he theorizes.

Dr. James P. Henry, professor of physiology at the University of Southern California School of Medicine, is deep in a long-term research project in which he is trying to discover more about hypertension and the effects of society on the individual.

"The history of hypertensive people," observes Dr. Henry,

"suggests that they usually have had difficult childhoods and they have grave difficulties in dealing with other people and in adapting to the realities of adult life."

Because it takes too long "to grow an adult human," Henry and his colleagues are observing what happens to a number of mouse colonies. The typical colony consists of about a dozen standard-size mouse boxes (each housing 6 to 8 mice), connected by a network of tubes just big enough for the mice to scoot around in but not big enough for them to pass each other.

A normal, socially adjusted colony is stocked by taking half a dozen pregnant females from a genetically pure strain of mice. The mothers are left to nurse their young, which are thus raised together as one big family.

When they can be weaned, at about three weeks, the mothers are removed and the total number of males and females limited to about 3 or 4 in a box. In this way, the whole colony has a maximum of residents allowing a reasonable amount of space.

In due course, the "socialized" mice set up house, elect boss mice, work out territories, have a separate latrine section, and a separate box for all subordinate males; the females raise the young contentedly in another box. In short, left in peace and quiet from birth, mice from the same environment have a spontaneous organization and live without signs of hypertension.

But what makes blood pressures rise? On the theory that people with hypertension usually have had difficult childhoods and have difficulties dealing with other people, Henry and his co-workers put mice in isolation in small jars from the instant they were weaned and before they had a chance to socialize. Then, at the age of 4 months they were placed with other mice that had been similarly isolated and were allowed to interact in an identical mouse city made up of interconnected boxes.

Henry found that hypertension develops as soon as these deprived mice are involved in social interaction. "Each male," he reports, "tries to be boss and they are constantly fighting. Few babies are born, and these never survive the first few days. The mice develop a persistent type of hypertension with an average pressure of about 160 millimeters of mercury."

In the many experiments conducted in the USC laboratory since the long-term study began, it has been found that the male's normal tendency to fight is greatly enhanced by mixing in some females. But if the males are castrated, everyone then settles down and pressures in such a mouse colony are lower than normal.

Fighting occurs and hypertension develops whenever males that are strange to each other are mixed in a box. Females may actually have a mild rise in pressure when caged with neutered males.

On one occasion, female pressures became elevated as a result of an accident. In removing the young of a colony to keep the population within bounds, one group lost all its young because all were well past weaning age. The adults showed increased blood pressures and fighting developed. One speculation is that the females were bereaved. The experiment is being repeated because the mothers later developed an unusually high number of breast tumors.

A recent experiment has studied the effects of caffeine, which is a brain stimulator. "Mice in a competitive society tend to get a bit more touchy as they get older, just like people," Dr. Henry says. "When we fed coffee to a group of normal sibling males that had just barely tolerated each other without serious conflict, fighting broke out."

Comparing this situation to human society, Henry suggests that an excess of coffee taken when an individual is already tense could make him more hostile in a group situation. "People vary in their ability to get along with others, of course. Some are phlegmatic by nature; others are terribly excitable. Each person should be aware of how he reacts, and it might be well for the easily stressed person to limit his intake of stimulants in the company of others."

Henry's belief is that much of the degenerative disease of today has social roots and prevention is probably more feasible than cure. He acknowledges that prevention might cost us something in our way of living. "It might mean slow-ing down the rate of progress. Progress means change; and change is one of the first enemies."

In addition to society's intense competitiveness and achievement motivation as a source of hypertension, Henry believes another source may be what he calls "male-female infighting." The togetherness of men and women may be stressful after long periods, he believes, and he points to the tendency of the sexes to congregate separately at social gatherings.

"There is," Henry observes, "no gross structural difference between the male and female brain but there is a big functional effect due to the male and female hormones. What is fundamental is that mammals have to play roles; there must be dominants and rivals—both male and female, nursing mothers and young, and subordinates of both sexes in order to make a viable mouse society. It is these social conventions that divide the available territory and stabilize the colony. It is the inability to accept the various roles that creates the problems in the disrupted society." And it would appear then that in the hypertension of mice as well as men, what matters is "the games people play."

6

When Cures Are Possible

Almost all hypertension, even the most severe, now can be controlled.

In the vast majority of cases, the hypertension is "essential," meaning that no known underlying physical abnormality can be pinpointed as the prime cause of the pressure elevation.

We will continue with the essential hypertension story— with the drug or other measures, sometimes simple, that can be used to bring such pressure elevation under effective control—in the following chapters.

In contrast to the many with essential hypertension, there is a small group of people with hypertension that can be traced to some definite physical cause. Often, such a cause can be corrected, and, when it is, the hypertension it has produced disappears.

In this chapter, we will consider the potentially curable forms of blood pressure elevation. And it is logical to do so here. For, although the numbers of people who have such hypertension may be relatively small, whenever anyone is newly diagnosed as a hypertensive, consideration is given to the possibility that there may be a curable abnormality before the patient is classified as having essential hypertension and treated for that.

PINCHING OF THE AORTA

The aorta, we have seen, is the body's major trunkline artery, big as a garden hose, emerging from the heart. From it, all the arteries carrying blood to all parts of the body branch off.

In a relatively few people, coarctation—or constriction—of the aorta is present from birth. The constriction or pinching may be minor, or it may be so great that only a pinpoint channel remains within the aorta at the site of pinching. Because of the pinching, the heart must work harder to push blood past the obstruction and blood pressure rises.

There may be no troublesome symptoms of any kind in the presence of coarctation of the aorta. But especially in children and young adults found to have hypertension, the problem may be suspected and checked for.

The tests are simple. The constriction usually occurs at a point in the aorta just beyond where the arteries carrying blood to the head and arms branch off. Though it takes high pressure to force blood past the obstruction, and this pressure is transmitted fully to the arteries going to the arms, the pressure is somewhat reduced by the time blood is past the obstruction and flowing to the leg arteries.

Thus, if blood pressure is high when measured as usual at the elbow but is much lower when measured over a leg artery, there is an immediate alert to the possibility of coarctation of the aorta.

If a patient has a significant degree of coarctation and is asked to jump up and down until out of breath, a marked increase in systolic blood pressure, sometimes to a level as high as 300, will be found in the arms immediately after the exercise. The physician may also check further by inspecting the back for pulsating arteries there and by looking for a notching of the ribs on the chest X ray.

Surgery usually can correct the coarctation and eliminate the hypertension. In the surgery, there is no need to go into the heart. The constricted segment of aorta is removed and the healthy portions remaining are then joined together. If the section that must be removed is extensive, a synthetic graft may be used between the healthy portions of the aorta. After a stay of about two weeks in the hospital, the patient often is ready to go home in good health.

PHEOCHROMOCYTOMA

Among the more common of the relatively rare causes of hypertension is a tumor, a pheochromocytoma, of an adrenal gland atop a kidney.

As noted earlier, the adrenal glands secrete hormones such as epinephrine, also known as adrenalin, and norepinephrine. These messenger substances help the body in emergency situations: they stimulate the heart, increase blood pressure, and aid in getting more blood to tissues, such as muscles, which may need it when the body has to fight or flee.

But overproduction of these hormones by the pheochromocytoma tumor can be responsible for hypertension. Most often the tumor is benign rather than cancerous, and cure usually follows its surgical removal.

Hypertension from a pheochromocytoma can occur at any age but tends to occur most often in young adults.

The symptoms are exactly like those which would be caused by injecting large amounts of epinephrine or norepinephrine or both. Norepinephrine, which primarily constricts blood vessels, does not have important other effects. But epinephrine, in addition to constricting vessels, increases body metabolism and produces marked sweating, flushing, and high blood-sugar levels. The symptoms will vary depending upon whether one substance or the other is predominantly secreted by the tumor. If epinephrine is predominant, there may be no alarming symptoms. If the major secretion is norepinephrine, hypertension may be associated with pounding headaches, nausea, palpitation, and faintness. There may be intolerance to heat, excessive sweating, and a flushed and anxious appearance.

With a pheochromocytoma, the blood pressure level may be either normal or elevated between attacks. The attacks may be triggered by emotional stress or by pressure over the tumor area. In one case, while a physician was examining the flank of a patient, the patient experienced an episode of pounding headache accompanied by nausea and perspiration and his blood pressure rose from normal levels to 280/140.

One of the older tests for pheochromocytoma, which still may be used on occasion, involves injecting small doses of a chemical, histamine. When histamine is injected into a vein of a normal person, it usually produces a drop in pressure for a short period and the fall is often associated with a flushing sensation. But in a patient with pheochromocytoma, the injection triggers the release of large quantities of hormones and pressure rises.

One of the newer tests makes use of a compound that has a specific antihormone action. When it is injected into a vein, the result is as might be expected. If the pressure elevation is caused by excess hormone secretion from a tumor, then the injection produces a temporary drop in pressure because of its antihormone activity. If the elevation is not related to excess adrenal hormones, there is no drop.

More recently, it has also become possible to measure in urine the products of the breakdown in the body of hormones secreted by a pheochromocytoma. One such product is vanillinemandelic acid. Large amounts of it can be found in the urine of patients whose hypertension is the result of a pheochromocytoma.

When such tests are positive, the pheochromocytoma can be located by X-ray studies and then can be removed surgically.

Typical of the value of such removal is the case of a 42-year-old man who had been suffering from pounding headaches, excessive nervousness. and excessive sweating for six months. His blood pressure was 190/110. Tests indicated a pheochromocytoma. Through an incision between the ribs, a 165-gram (almost 6 ounce) tumor was removed from the right adrenal gland. His blood pressure came down to normal and his symptoms disappeared promptly.

Another patient had been experiencing severe headaches, shortness of breath, and excessive sweating for several years. His blood pressure was 172/115. After he tested positive for a pheochromocytoma, a 185-gram tumor was removed from the right adrenal gland. His blood pressure promptly fell to 140/95. It has remained there for three years thus far and he has been free of symptoms.

ALDOSTERONISM

This is another adrenal gland disorder that may cause hypertension.

Adolsterone is a substance that increases salt retention in the body and raises blood pressure through a complicated chemical derangement.

In aldosteronism, there is abnormal secretion of aldosterone. Sometimes the problem stems from a kidney blood vessel condition, which in itself may produce hypertension and which also may stimulate the adrenal gland to produce excess amounts of aldosterone, complicating the hypertension still further. In such cases, the kidney blood vessel condition requires treatment.

But aldosteronism, a form called primary aldosteronism, may result from a small adrenal gland adenoma, or tumor. Usually, primary aldosteronism is associated with only moderate elevation of pressure. Classical symptoms include muscular weakness, headache, numbness and pricking sensations, excessive urine secretion, and excessive thirst. But few or no such symptoms may be present.

Primary aldosteronism is rare. Several tests may be used to check for the condition. Most patients will excrete a dilute alkaline urine. When a patient with primary aldosteronism is given one of the drugs often used in treating essential hypertension, a telltale indication may be a fall in the level of potassium in the blood. When such tests suggest aldosteronism, other more direct tests to check on the actual secretion rates of aldosterone can be made.

Once it is clear that a patient has primary aldosteronism, the responsible tumor can be removed surgically. Rarely is it malignant and its removal often results in complete disappearance of hypertension and any symptoms that have stemmed from it.

CUSHING'S SYNDROME

Another uncommon cause of hypertension is called Cushing's syndrome after the great neurosurgeon Harvey Cushing.

Here again the problem lies with excessive adrenal gland secretions. In addition to elevated blood pressure, there may be obesity, muscle weakness, easy bruising, thinning of the bones. Kidney stones and diabetes may occur. Psychiatric disturbances are common. Women usually have menstrual irregularities.

The adrenal glands are under the control of the pituitary gland at the base of the brain in the center of the head. In some cases, excess adrenal activity may be caused by a pituitary gland tumor which secretes large amounts of a hormone that stimulates the adrenal glands. Another possible cause may be an adrenal gland tumor.

Various tests can be used in the diagnosis of Cushing's syndrome. Blood tests may reveal abnormal levels of adrenal hormone. So may urine tests. Other chemical tests can help determine whether an adrenal gland tumor or a pituitary tumor is involved. In some cases, a pituitary tumor may press against the base of the skull and produce a deformity that can be recognized on X rays of the head.

Often, surgery to remove an adrenal gland tumor, or supervoltage irradiation treatment of a pituitary gland tumor, will bring great benefits, lowering the blood pressure and relieving muscle weakness and other symptoms.

INFECTIONS

Chronic, long-continued infection of the kidneys may produce hypertension. Such an infection may arise from repeated infections elsewhere in the urinary tract. Finally, the kidneys may be invaded and kidney function may be reduced, with subsequent elevation of blood pressure.

In some cases, intensive treatment with antibacterials may overcome a chronic infection, and hypertension may be cured. When this is not possible, the hypertension still may be controlled effectively by the type of drug treatment used for essential hypertension.

Urinary tract infections are often silent, producing no warning symptoms. But their presence can be determined by urine tests revealing abnormal numbers of bacteria, and physicians today are alert to the need for intensive treatment when symptomless infections are discovered.

KIDNEY ARTERY HYPERTENSION

Disease of a kidney artery is one of the most common curable causes of hypertension. The disease may occur at any age. In youth it may result from abnormal growth of a portion of a kidney artery wall; in older age, from atherosclerotic plaques. It may occur in both major kidney arteries although it usually affects one kidney more than the other.

Whether as the result of abnormal artery-wall growth or of the fatty deposits of atherosclerosis, the artery bore is diminished and blood flow through it is disturbed. Rebelling against the diminished flow, the kidney releases a substance, renin, into the blood. The substance triggers formation of aldosterone, which raises blood pressure.

Renovascular hypertension, as kidney artery-produced blood pressure elevation is called, can be diagnosed with the aid of various tests. For example, one laboratory procedure, called the intravenous pyelogram, involves injecting dye, which is painless, into a vein in the arm. The dye circulates to the kidneys and sharpens X-ray pictures that are taken over the kidney area to help in the diagnosis. Also, kidney areas may be scanned after the injection of harmless doses of radioactive material, a procedure that can be carried out in the doctor's office.

Renovascular hypertension often can be cured by surgery. In some cases, the interior of the obstructed section of artery may be cleaned out; in others, the diseased section may be removed and the healthy portions joined; in still others, a graft may be used to bypass the obstructed section.

Renovascular hypertension also can be controlled in many cases by drug treatment.

Since there are two alternatives—surgical and medical treatment—many factors may be considered before one or the other is chosen.

One factor is the type of narrowing of the artery. As a group, patients with atherosclerotic narrowing—fatty deposits that produce the blocking—generally do not benefit as much from surgery as do those with nonatherosclerotic narrowing. Also important is the extent of the narrowing. When a small portion of a kidney artery is affected, surgery is much more feasible.

Age is also a factor. Most young hypertensives with kidney artery disease are basically healthy and can withstand surgery better and have more potential for improvement.

Even half a dozen years ago, when surgeons at Baylor University Medical School reported results of surgery in 600 patients of all ages, they could point to the fact that over-all about half had benefitted with return to normal blood pressure whereas many others had reduced pressures. Of those operated on five or more years before, 75 percent were alive, 80 percent had shown improvement, and half had normal pressure.

Currently, based on experience at major medical centers, a young person with a nonatherosclerotic obstruction of a kidney artery has, with successful surgery, a 70 to 80 percent chance of being cured of hypertension for a lifetime. For an elderly patient with an atherosclerotic obstruction, surgery offers about a 50 percent chance of permanent cure of the hypertension.

When surgical treatment does not seem feasible, medical treatment usually is effective. Several years ago, there was a feeling that renovascular hypertension is more resistant to drug treatment than is essential hypertension, but subsequent experience has shown that this is not the fact. In most cases, it is now known, pressure can be reduced to normal or very near normal levels and maintained at such levels for years.

HOW MANY TESTS?

Only a small percentage of hypertensive patients have curable hypertension.

Beyond use of careful, thorough physical examination, we have seen that there are many laboratory techniques and specialized procedures that can be used to uncover the curable forms: test doses of various drugs; special tests of blood and urine; special tests to determine the way each of the two kidneys is functioning; special X-ray studies of the kidney arteries with the aid of dyes that make them clearly visible; and still others.

Some of the tests entail considerable expense. To use them routinely in every hypertensive patient may be impractical. The physician must use the best possible judgment in determining those patients in whom a curable type of hypertension is most likely to be found and what tests may be particularly useful.

There is no one-and-one-only approved approach.

Often, only a few relatively simple tests may be needed. They may include measurement of blood pressure in the legs to detect coarctation of the aorta. A chest X ray may also show notching of the ribs as an indication of coarctation. The level of potassium in the blood is useful in detecting primary aldosteronism. Pheochromocytoma may be suspected if a patient is thin, complains of frequent headaches and palpitations, and the diagnosis may be confirmed by a urine test. Often the patient with hypertension caused by Cushing's syndrome has a characteristic appearance such as a moon-faced look, that alerts the physician.

When it comes to renovascular hypertension, because most patients over the age of 50 will be treated medically rather than surgically, many good physicians believe that only patients above 50 who do not respond well to drug treatment may need intensive tests for kidney artery disease.

7

Control Without Drugs

Jack Norm married a girl who pleased him in many ways. She was beautiful; she was intelligent; and she had a great zest for cooking. In college, he had been lean and tough, no varsity athlete but a good man with basketball, baseball, tennis racket, and golf club.

In his bachelor days, he ate well but not extravagantly, and kept in vigorous trim with tennis, golf, and handball as well. When he married, he had a full home life, less time for sports, and the meals were delectable.

His hypertension showed up during a routine physical examination when he was 36. By then he was hardly lean. He had stored up a lot of calories in his eight years of marriage. His blood pressure was 165/101. His weight was 28 pounds over what it had been in his college and bachelor days.

"There are pills to bring down the blood pressure," his doctor told him. "But you may not need them. If you slim down—which you ought to do anyhow for a lot of reasons besides your blood pressure—the pressure may well come down without pills."

Up to here there is nothing unusual in Jack's story—the loss of fitness and leanness, the steady gain in fat in the late twenties and early thirties. Many men go through that; so do many women.

Jack didn't lose his excess poundage overnight, or in a month or two. He made no effort to do that. He went on no stringent diet. He pushed back a bit earlier from the table; he ate everything but a bit less of it; he gradually bucked up

93

his physical activity with walks, runs, and, later, a couple of handball sessions a week during his lunch hours.

He lost about a pound a week. By the time he had lost half a dozen pounds, his blood pressure showed a little fall. When he was down to his old and fit weight, his blood pressure was normal.

That was three years ago, and he hasn't regained any weight and his blood pressure has stayed normal.

And that is what makes Jack's story unusual, not that his hypertension melted away with the excess body lard but that he managed to lose weight sensibly, get down to proper weight successfully, and stay there.

There is no shortage today of effective drugs for hypertension. There are many. Often they are required and significantly elevated pressure cannot be normalized without them. But sometimes the response to drugs can be greatly improved, and lesser amounts of them may be needed, when some basic measures are used. And sometimes the need for drugs may be avoided completely with the use of such basic measures, of which loss of excess weight is one.

THE HEAVINESS BURDEN

We've already seen that excess weight is commonly accompanied by an increase in blood pressure. As body weight increases, so does the volume of blood. Fatty tissue, like any other tissue, must be supplied with blood. It has been estimated that each extra pound of fat requires about a mile of capillaries to feed it. Thus, in overweight people the heart has to pump more blood through a more extensive blood vessel system, increasing its burden.

If a patient with hypertension is distinctly obese, most physicians would do everything possible to encourage him to take off excess weight. Many would encourage even those moderately overweight to reduce as an important first step, perhaps the only necessary step, in treatment.

"The association between obesity and hypertension is unequivocal. The single most important factor related to risk of hypertension is overweight—at least the single most important factor amenable to environmental influence," observes Dr. Jeremiah Stamler, professor and chairman of Northwestern University Medical School's Department of Community Health and Preventive Medicine.

In addition to its association with hypertension (Chapter 5), which alone would make it important enough, excess weight can contribute in other ways to excessive death rates.

When it comes to individual diseases, insurance actuarial tables show that, as compared with the general population, men and women who are overweight have, respectively, these mortality excesses: 142 and 175 percent for heart attacks; 149 and 162 percent for cerebral hemorrhage; 191 and 212 percent for chronic nephritis (kidney disease); 168 and 211 percent for liver and gallbladder cancer; 383 and 372 percent for diabetes; 249 and 147 percent for cirrhosis of the liver; 154 and 141 percent for hernia and intestinal obstruction.

Thus, for any person who is hypertensive and overweight, weight reduction, if it can be accomplished sensibly, successfully, and permanently, has much to recommend it.

Unhappily, weight reduction efforts generally rank high in frustration and anxiety. A lot of people spend a lot of time futilely trying to reduce.

To no small extent, the futility stems from a desire for the quick and easy way, the reach for the latest panacea, the failure to come to grips with the basic problem—that obesity results from an intake of more calories than are needed to meet energy needs. The corollary, of course, is that if excess weight is to be lost, fewer calories must be taken in than are needed for energy, which provides the opportunity for the stored calories to be used up.

Many drugs have been tried for treating obesity, without proof of lasting benefit. Thyroid, effective and safe only in people with thyroid deficiency (a very small fraction of the obese), has been used for others without effect. Pituitary-like hormones have been employed, without benefit. Digitalis to induce appetite loss can be extremely risky and there is no likelihood of permanent benefit in terms of weight loss.

Amphetamines depress appetite only for a few weeks and most people quickly become tolerant; if they keep increasing the dose to get the same effect as they once did with lesser doses, they may get toxic effects, experience mental disturbances, and become psychically dependent on the drugs.

Crash diets (new ones turn up with great regularity) that bring down weight with startling suddenness—accomplishing great losses in short periods—may do more harm than good. They impose a strain. More than that, they do not provide any reasonable way to maintain weight loss, once it is achieved. Almost invariably, the crash dieter is an endlessly repetitive dieter. Quick loss is followed by quick gain.

There may be a danger many people do not realize in crash on-again-off-again dieting. Studies show that increased deposits of cholesterol may be laid down on artery walls during periods of weight gain. No studies indicate that the deposits are melted away during periods of weight loss. To go through repetitive periods of weight loss and weight gain, with increased deposition of cholesterol during the gain periods, may be only to increase the risks of atherosclerotic arteries.

It is much more sensible to balance calorie intake with energy needs. A calorie is a measure of the energy-producing value of food. Some foods have many calories and provide much energy; some have few calories and provide relatively little. Energy is used—calories are consumed—in many ways: just lying in bed or sitting quietly consumes some; working at a desk uses up some. The more vigorous an activity, the greater the calorie consumption.

It takes 3,500 calories to make a pound of fat. If you were to maintain your present level of activity and simply ate just 100 fewer calories a day, you would lose a pound in 35 days. Not startling. But then cutting out only 100 calories a day is not demanding. You can live with it. It imposes no great hardships. In a few days, you hardly miss that extra slice of bread or that extra slop of cream in some of your cups of coffee, or anything else representing 100 calories.

A pound in 35 days doesn't seem like much. But it adds up

in a year to more than 10 pounds. And that is 10 pounds off with a good chance of keeping them permanently off.

It is hardly necessary, of course, to limit weight reduction to a rate of 10 pounds a year. You may want to, and be able to, double or triple that rate.

And you may be able to do so all the more readily, without experiencing pangs of hunger or even feelings of deprivation, if you couple a reasonable calorie cutdown with a reasonable calorie-expenditure increase. See the tables, including the table for calorie expenditure, in the Appendix.

Before getting into the subject of exercise—as an aid not only in reducing weight but possibly, also, as a direct aid in reducing elevated pressure—another aspect of eating deserves mention.

THE CHOLESTEROL QUESTION

Is it necessary to avoid cholesterol-rich foods?

As we know, cholesterol has been linked with atherosclerosis, the fatty, artery-clogging deposits that may set the stage for heart attacks, strokes, and kidney trouble. Hypertension may help to drive those deposits in, and control of hypertension can be expected to help greatly in controlling atherosclerosis.

Still, obviously, it would not do to rest content with controlling one factor if another can be controlled without great difficulty.

Some foods are very rich in cholesterol. These include egg yolk, butter, shrimp, kidney, sweetbreads, and brains. (A full listing is included in the Appendix.) Moderation in their intake can help—unless your physician because of your actual blood cholesterol levels suggests almost complete avoidance.

The body manufactures its own cholesterol too. And certain fatty foods lend themselves well to the making of excess body production of cholesterol. These are the saturated fats found in butter, whole milk, and many meats (particularly beef, lamb, and pork).

The American diet, with its heavily marbled meats, its fat-laden snacks and drinks, has become much too fatty in the opinion of many leading nutritional authorities as well as physicians concerned with heart disease and strokes. All of us might do well to moderate total fat intake.

Moderation in all fat intake should be kept in mind when you hear discussions of the merits of simply substituting unsaturated fats for the saturated. Unsaturated fats are the "soft" fats, such as those contained in vegetable oils, fish and fowl, and many margarines. True, there is evidence that, in terms of cholesterol levels in the blood, a change in the ratio of saturated and unsaturated fat intake—in favor of less saturated and more unsaturated—is beneficial.

But from an overall standpoint, in terms not only of cholesterol-level reduction but of weight reduction as well, the best bet may be not to depend merely upon changing a ratio but also on moderating the total dietary use of fats.

SALT IN YOUR DIET

At one point, as we have seen earlier, there was little else that could be done to help many hypertensives beyond rigid limitation of salt intake.

The famed rice diet of some years ago was an extreme low-salt diet. Patients had to use measured amounts of rice, tomatoes, fruit juice, and vitamins, and nothing else. There was no magic in the rice, tomatoes, fruit juices, or vitamins; they simply lacked salt. There are not many such foods.

If salt is almost completely removed from the diet, blood pressure is very likely to fall. But almost complete removal of salt is not easy to accomplish, nor to live with.

The average U.S. salt intake is about 15 grams a day. Severe restriction meant limiting intake to 200 milligrams —2/10 of a gram—a day. Most physicians now agree that a very low salt diet has become an archaic form of treatment with the availability of modern diuretic drugs, which, as we will see later, can control salt.

But moderate restriction of salt may be desirable. Your

physician may suggest limiting salt intake to something on the order of about 5 grams a day. That could allow use of a modest amount of salt for cooking purposes but a much reduced use of salt at the table and avoidance of very salty foods such as crackers, potato chips, and pretzels, as indicated in the salt-content tables in the Appendix.

EXERCISE TO AID WEIGHT REDUCTION— AND HYPERTENSION CONTROL

Go out and engage in some very vigorous physical activity every week or so—a hard game of handball or tennis, for example—and it is not likely that it will help you lose weight. It is likely that your appetite will increase; it may well impose a strain you should not have to bear and cannot tolerate well. It may, in fact, be bad for your heart.

Moderate exercise is a different matter. If, for example, you start with a moderately paced walk of half a mile, or a mile, once a day, you'll get no severe muscular pain and you're not likely to note any marked increase in appetite. Nor will your appetite be likely to increase as you step up the pace gradually, walking a little faster and progressively greater distances.

You will be expending more calories but imposing no sudden excessive demands on your body, nor stimulating your appetite.

Unless you have some special condition your physician finds calls for limiting your activity, you can, with a reasonable physical effort, help lose weight, control your hypertension, and improve your health.

The values of exercise, as demonstrated by scores of studies, are, indeed, many.

The relationship between exercise and weight has been shown repeatedly. Subjects, all young men, were offered payment if they could keep their weight constant. At first the men were placed on a low-calorie diet. They soon found they had to restrict their physical activities to keep their weight stationary. Then the diet was moved way up, to 6,000 calories a day. Now they had to exercise more vigorously than ever, running, rowing, doing calisthenics, to hold their weight steady.

The ability of exercise to keep blood cholesterol levels in check has also been shown in many studies. When, for example, a group of more than 100 Marines in vigorous training were fed upward of 4,500 calories a day and the diet was deliberately made heavy with fat and continued for six months, the men still had unchanged blood fat levels and weight at the end of the study because of continuous hard physical activity. In a Harvard study, medical students were put to exercising vigorously while their caloric intake was doubled. As long as they remained physically active, their weight and blood fat levels remain unchanged. Soon after exercising stopped, both weight and blood fats shot up.

Many studies also suggest beneficial effects of exercise on the heart muscle, and on the blood circulation to the heart. With exercise, any muscle, the biceps on your arm, for example, can be expected to become stronger, more efficient, able to take loads for longer periods with less fatigue.

Similarly, the well-trained heart muscle becomes more efficient. It can pump more blood with less effort. For example, the first 4-minute miler, Roger Bannister (now a physician), had, originally, an average heart rate in the mid-70s when sitting still or resting. After training for his record run, his resting heart rate dropped to 40 beats a minute. His heart could pump more blood with each beat, and needed fewer beats to supply body needs.

There is also evidence that exercise stimulates collateral circulation for the heart muscle. As we've seen, the coronary artery system we are endowed with consists of two great coronary arteries and their branches. Experiments have demonstrated that with exercise, additional branches and interconnections are laid down. With exercise, the heart muscle calls for more blood and nutrition, and the body responds by adding collaterals. They can come in handy. If a coronary artery or a main branch should become blocked by disease, collaterals—spare vessels—sometimes can quickly take over the job of rerouting blood around the blocked vessel, avoiding a heart attack. Moreover, collaterals may explain why some people, despite severe narrowing of their major coronary arteries, never experience angina, or chest pain. In their cases, fortunately, collateral growth seems to have kept pace with the progress of atherosclerosis, and the collaterals have kept the heart muscle from suffering blood deprivation.

Actually, some physicians today use carefully controlled exercises in patients with angina and even in patients who have suffered heart attacks in an effort to stimulate the formation of collaterals to help overcome the angina and help reduce the likelihood of another heart attack.

THE EFFECT OF EXERCISE
ON BLOOD PRESSURE

Studies suggest that exercise may be of value in keeping blood pressure at normal levels and in bringing about some reduction of elevated pressure.

Sixty-one former champion runners and cross-country skiers, aged 40 to 79, were examined and compared with nonathletes of the same ages. Whereas mean blood pressures for the nonathletes were above normal, those for the athletes were within normal limits.

According to reports from the Soviet Union, half of all endurance athletes there listed as "Masters of Sport" have systolic blood pressures of 99 or less, well below the 140 upper limit of normal.

In one experiment at the San Diego State College Exercise Laboratory, 23 hypertensive men were placed on a program of moderate exercise consisting of 15 to 20 minutes of warm-up calisthenics plus no more than 35 minutes of walking-jogging twice a week. After six months of the program, their mean blood pressure had fallen from 159/105 to 146/93.

In another study with 105 urban men, aged 25 to 60, Dr. George V. Mann and his associates at Vanderbilt University School of Medicine and the Department of Physical Education of George Peabody College for Teachers, Nashville,

Tennessee, sought to find a feasible system of supervised exercise and to measure the effects on heart disease risk factors.

The 105 men included professionals, white- and blue-collar workers, and a few laborers. They were asked to attend at least 4 of 5 weekly training sessions, either from 6 A.M. to 7 A.M. or from 5 P.M. to 6 P.M. The training was always carried out in groups led by an instructor and consisted of calisthenics and alternate periods of walking, jogging, and running. Each man was assigned to one of three levels of exercise intensity according to his medical history, physical examination, and initial fitness. Men were promoted to higher intensity levels as their proficiency increased.

The program lasted six months and 76 percent of the men stuck with it. At the end, 96 percent of the men said they would do it again.

There was marked improvement in feelings of fitness, including a significant improvement in weight. Blood cholesterol levels came down, without dietary restrictions. And blood pressures fell significantly.

After a thorough analysis of the results, Dr. Mann and his colleagues concluded that only three training sessions a week are really needed to produce measurable benefits, and that benefits often can be maintained with as little as one training session a week, requiring no more than 30 minutes.

How do some leading heart and hypertension specialists feel about exercise for hypertensive patients?

At a recent symposium on hypertension, members of a distinguished panel had these comments to make.

Said Dr. Edward Freis, Lasker Award winner for his Veterans Administration studies on hypertension treatment: "I think it is important that the patient be encouraged to exercise, to take any kind of physical exercise within the limits of his capability in regard to symptoms. He can exercise up to tolerance. If he does not have cardiac [heart] complications with his hypertension, there is no reason why he should not, unless he is taking certain antihypertensive drugs which produce hypotensive collapse [very low blood pressure] with violent exercise."

Dr. Harriet P. Dustan of the Cleveland Clinic: "Yes, I advise them to exercise regularly. It is impressive how sedentary and inactive most of our patients are now. I discuss with them their exercise patterns or lack thereof and their distaste for exercise, because this is very real. Sometimes, even walking upstairs becomes unpleasant because of continued inactivity and will be avoided whenever possible. This also applies to the general population."

If you have hypertension, your physician may well have some specific advice on exercise, its possible value as an aid in controlling your blood pressure without the need for drugs, or for making it easier to control with drugs, and its possible values for you in other ways. He may have specific advice as to kind of exercise, how to begin, and how to progress. No person who has long been sedentary is well advised to undertake an exercise program without medical evaluation and advice. That is certainly true for the person who has hypertension.

SMOKING

Hypertension can be controlled in cigarette smokers. Giving up the smoking habit is not, by any means, an absolute requirement for bringing blood pressure elevations down to normal.

But most physicians now counsel hypertensive patients to make an effort to give up cigarettes and, if they do not wish to stop smoking entirely, to switch to pipe or cigar.

One of the striking facts that have come out of the Framingham studies is that cigarette smoking is the most impressive single additive, much more so even than elevated blood fats, for increasing the risk of heart attack and stroke for the person who has hypertension.

For some years now, of course, cigarettes have had a "bad press." Their association with lung cancer, chronic bronchitis, and emphysema has been well publicized. An association between cigarettes and other diseases has also been documented by many studies. The diseases include cancer of the larynx, cancer of the esophagus, cancer of the urinary bladder, and peptic ulcer.

Less well publicized has been the association of cigarette smoking with diseases of the blood vessels and the heart.

Cigarette smoking stimulates the adrenal glands, which release excess amounts of hormones. This release causes an increase in free fatty acids in the blood observed upon the inhalation of cigarette smoke.

For both smokers and nonsmokers, the risk of dying from coronary heart disease increases with increasing blood pressure, and the risk is higher among smokers than among nonsmokers at every level of blood pressure. Thus, cigarette smoking increases coronary heart disease mortality independently of its effect on blood pressure and of the effect of hypertension on coronary heart disease.

Cigarette smoking, by stimulating the adrenals, causes an increased heart rate and increases the tension of the heart muscle, and in both ways adds to the work of the heart and the need for oxygen and other nutrients. Yet, at the same time, the smoking interferes with increased blood flow and oxygen supply to the heart. For one thing, by interfering with lung function, cigarette smoking may reduce the amount of oxygen that can be carried in the blood to the heart muscle.

For another, cigarette smoke contains carbon monoxide. When the carbon monoxide is inhaled, it gets into the blood and usurps the place of oxygen there, so less oxygen is available to the tissues, including the heart muscle.

Thus, while it is not essential to give up cigarettes in order to bring hypertension under control, giving them up may help to simplify control, and, beyond that, eliminate the risk-increasing effects cigarettes have independently of their effects on blood pressure.

Certainly, most physicians now will not insist that a hypertensive patient abandon cigarettes. But they want the patient to have the known facts and the opportunity to make his own decision.

Moreover, not only have more and more physicians themselves given up cigarettes successfully, they report that more and more patients are able to do so.

Kicking the habit is certainly not easy for everyone. But it has been found to be much easier for some than long supposed.

Some studies suggest that there are four types of smokers. The *habitual* smoker is one who is hardly aware that he has a cigarette in his mouth; he smokes automatically; and the first step for such a smoker is to become aware of when he is smoking, to look hard at his pattern of smoking.

For the *positive affect* smoker, cigarettes may serve as either stimulant or relaxant; he enjoys handling a cigarette or the sight of smoke curling out of his mouth. The positive affect smoker, if he can persuade himself to make the effort, may find giving up cigarettes relatively easy.

The *negative affect* smoker uses cigarettes to relieve feelings of fear, distress, disgust, or shame. He may not smoke much or at all when things go well, when he is on vacation, or at a party, but when he is under tension he reaches for a cigarette. Such a smoker often can give up smoking with relative ease, and may stay away from it, if, when tense, he resorts to a strong substitute, such as nibbling on gingerroot.

The *addictive smoker* is one who is aware of any time he is not smoking. Although he may enjoy a cigarette only briefly, if at all, he is uncomfortable without one. For him, giving up smoking is not easy. Tapering off smoking may work for a few addictive smokers; some find it effective to quit cold, but first before doing so, to double their smoking, forcing themselves to smoke until they revolt against the increased dose of tar and nicotine and other smoke ingredients, and then quitting.

Smokers trying to quit have long resorted to chewing gum, sucking candy mints, nibbling on fruits and raw vegetables, but recent experience suggests that deep breathing from time to time may be as helpful or even more so, and that exercise also is helpful.

For those who want to stop but find it difficult or impossible to do on their own, group sessions are now available in many communities.

For those who have made efforts in the past to stop smoking, all of which failed, it is still quite possible to succeed.

A useful booklet, "If You Want to Give Up Cigarettes," published by the American Cancer Society, which can be obtained from a local chapter of the organization, is full of practical suggestions coming from many experimental stop-smoking programs.

For those who must smoke, choose cigarettes with less tar and nicotine. Avoid smoking them all the way down. The last third of a cigarette produces twice as much nicotine and tar as the first third; let it be. Take fewer puffs on each cigarette. Reduce inhaling.

Pipes and cigars are not entirely free of risk, but the disparity in the death rates between pipe and cigar smokers and those who smoke cigarettes suggests that there might be much saving of life and health if cigarette smokers unable to give up smoking entirely were to change to pipes and cigars.

COMBATING STRESS

There has been some tendency to think that all stress is bad. It isn't. Playing a game of tennis is stressful. So is watching a suspense thriller. Invariably, there is stress in life. Only when the stress is excessive and prolonged does it cause trouble.

Much has been said about the terrible stresses of modern living. But every generation has had its stresses. "There were stresses of the Wars of the Roses," says Dr. Irvine H. Page. "And it must have been pretty stressful trying to build a pyramid in ancient times. The Mayan Indians might have had their heads cut off or been made human sacrifices just because they happened to be on the losing soccer team, and this must have been a pretty stressful situation."

There has been a tendency to think of certain jobs as being excessively stressful. The greater the responsibility, it has been supposed, the greater the stress. A typical business executive has been supposed to be a hard driver, under constant stress, pressure ridden. But this may not necessarily be true at all—for example, among 270,000 Bell System employees in different jobs and at different levels of achievement, no relationship could be found indicating that men with the greatest responsibility suffered more from the effects of stress.

All of us experience stress; some of us handle it more effectively than others.

How may the handling of it be improved?

Stress often may be at least tempered if a deliberate attempt is made to interrupt it periodically. Any distraction —a book, movie, or a bit of physical activity—can be helpful.

Given insight into the havoc long-continued stress may create, some people are able to adjust to stressful conditions by deciding they will simply do their best and, having done so, refuse to worry and become unduly anxious.

Some who believe their work too stressful may try shifting to other work. But there are those who, accurately assessing the problem, find that much of their job stress stems from personality clashes with others, usually superiors, and that they can minimize the stress and get along better with an unpleasant superior by considering him a stress-driven person who may deserve sympathy rather than hate.

Physical activity is a help for many people in combating stress. Beyond the distraction it offers, physical activity also provides a healthy outlet for stress. Under stress, the body churns. Glandular activity surges so as to mobilize energy, to ready the body for action. It helps to use up the mobilized energy by physical activity instead of having it go swirling around within, with no outlet other than to create tension and trouble.

8

The Drug Story

The time was just after World War II. The patient was a physician himself. He had malignant hypertension; his diastolic blood pressure was 160; the situation was desperate. He had hoped that the nerve-cutting operation, sympathectomy, might help him. But already his kidney damage was extremely severe and the operation could not be performed.

At that time, no drug of any significant value in reducing severely elevated pressure was available.

But a discovery was made in connection with pentaquine, an antimalarial drug. In evaluating the drug, it had been necessary to consider not only its effectiveness against malaria but its safety as well. The drug was administered to a group of normal healthy volunteers, and it was noted then that in these men, after several days of doses higher than those actually used for malaria, their blood pressures fell from normal levels to abnormally low ones.

Could pentaquine be useful against hypertension? When it was tested on hypertensive patients, it did indeed lower pressure, but the doses needed led to serious side effects that prevented its use as an antihypertensive agent.

Still, with nothing else to be done for the physician with malignant hypertension who was rapidly progressing toward death, it seemed worthwhile to try pentaquine. On large doses, his blood pressure fell from 160 diastolic to 100. His headache disappeared, and so did the signs of congestive heart failure.

"This," recalls Dr. Edward Freis who treated him, "was the first time we had seen reversal of the signs of malignant hypertension following an antihypertensive drug. It was a most exciting experience and it convinced us of the value of the chemotherapeutic approach. Unfortunately, the patient's kidney failure gradually worsened, and he died several months later. However, his final months of life were more comfortable than they would have been without penta-quine."

Dr. Freis and other investigators, now greatly encouraged, hopefully looked for leads to other potentially useful drugs.

Veratrum, a medicinal herb, had been used for various purposes by American Indians. And in the nineteenth century physicians had used it to "soften" the pulse and lower body temperature in infections.

Freis and others found that veratrum could reduce pressure in hypertensive patients when injected into a vein. They were encouraged, too, because the blood flow and filtering capacity of the kidneys were not affected adversely, indicating that if hypertension could be treated successfully, the kidneys could adjust to the fall in pressure. Moreover, after injection of veratrum into hypertensive patients with congestive heart failure, there was dramatic evidence of clearing of the heart failure and improvement in the functioning of the heart.

But veratrum was a long way from being an ideal anti-hypertensive agent. Patients at times would develop unexpected severe reactions, with violent retching, sweating, and collapse. The attacks were brief, but they made the drug unacceptable for any but the most severe, life-threatening cases of hypertension.

Meanwhile, the rice diet had come into wide use. It was effective because of its extremely low salt content—less than 200 milligrams a day. It turned out that when the rice diet was combined with veratrum, many patients responded even better to the drug. Moreover, veratrum also turned out to be helpful in patients who had failed to respond to sympathectomy.

This showed that a combined attack on hypertension might be useful. By combining sympathectomy, a low salt diet, and veratrum, each acting through a different mechanism, it was sometimes possible to bring hypertension under control in patients who failed to respond to any single measure.

These were among the early pioneering efforts that were to lead to the drugs now available which allow physicians to control hypertension of all degrees of severity.

They are drugs that act in various ways. They include drugs that, ingeniously, are designed to relax the arterioles, the tiny pressure-controlling blood vessels, by various mechanisms. They include drugs that, in effect, perform chemical sympathectomy, surgery by chemical action, rather than by scalpel severing. They have the advantage not only of avoiding the need for actual surgery; chemical surgery is also reversible at any time simply by stopping the administration of a drug. Moreover, chemical surgery permits more precise control because drugs may reach areas the surgeon cannot penetrate.

CHEMICAL SURGERY DRUGS

Among the first of the new modern breed of effective antihypertensive drugs were powerful ganglionic blocking agents, which, in effect, performed chemical surgery.

The tiny arterioles, which relax and constrict affecting blood pressure, do so, as noted in Chapter 3, under nervous control. The nervous system that controls their activity, the sympathetic nervous system, has junction centers. The sympathetic nerves stretch from the midbrain down the spinal cord, and they branch off at various vertebrae. As they branch off, they enter the junction centers, called ganglia.

In a sense, a ganglion is much like the telephone terminal box found in any home. In the box, telephone wires from a switchboard or central telephone station come in and terminate. But there is also provision for the user to insert a male plug connected to a telephone. With plug in place, the telephone is ready for use.

In a ganglion, the nerve fibers from the spinal cord enter

and terminate. But also in the ganglion are nerve fibers which, from there, extend to the arterioles some distance away in the body. Between the ends of the nerve fibers from the spinal cord and the ends of those reaching to the arterioles is a space, called a synapse.

But in this situation, there is no plug to connect the fibers so that messages can flow. Instead, a nerve impulse bridges the space, or synapse, by means of a chemical reaction, a kind of chemical messenger service.

But ganglionic blocking agents obstruct the messenger service; they interfere with the chemical reaction. Thus, excessive sympathetic nervous impulses acting to keep the arterioles constricted and the blood pressure up are dampened, and the arterioles can relax.

Actually, tests made as far back as 1899 showed that nicotine had this blocking effect, but was too poisonous to be used in the amounts needed.

A number of potentially useful blocking agents were also tried after World War II by American investigators. One was tetraethylammonium but it was found to have too brief an action to be of value in treating hypertension. Other test agents also had proved impractical for one reason or another.

Then, in 1950, British investigators began to report successful treatment of malignant hypertension with a new blocking agent, hexamethonium. And soon investigators in this country were confirming that it was the first useful blocking agent. It was longer acting than previous drugs and produced greater blockage. It had some drawbacks: it had to be injected several times a day and it sometimes produced side effects such as blurring of vision, dry mouth, and constipation. It was valuable for severe hypertension but, beyond that, had limited usefulness.

By now, however, many pharmaceutical companies had entered into the search for more effective antihypertensive agents.

Another ganglionic blocking agent that followed, chlorisondamine, produced a longer, smoother response with fewer undesirable side effects.

And soon many other new drugs with different modes of action became available for testing.

THE RELAXERS

Actually, almost at the same time that the first blockers were being developed and studied, another type of drug, hydralazine, emerged. Instead of acting in the ganglia, hydralazine appears to act directly on the muscle walls of blood vessels, relaxing them.

Hydralazine produced a more gradual and more lasting fall in pressure than the ganglionic blockers. It also increased blood flow to the kidneys, and since decreased flow to the kidneys is a known source of hypertension, the increased flow with hydralazine was considered desirable.

When used alone, hydralazine sometimes was not effective unless given in high doses, which then might produce undesirable effects. Soon, however, a combination of small amounts of hydralazine and hexamethonium was proving helpful.

Very quickly came another important new agent, reserpine, a drug purified from the Indian plant, *rauwolfia serpentina*. The powdered root of *rauwolfia* had been used in India for centuries as a medicinal herb for treating the mentally disturbed. Then an Indian heart specialist reported that it seemed to be effective in hypertension. Soon studies in this country were confirming the observation and, before long, reserpine, the pure active ingredient of *rauwolfia*, became available. The Appendix lists the various trade names of antihypertensive drugs.

Reserpine was the first drug to which the term "tranquilizer" was applied. It acts calmatively in the central nervous system. In doing that, it may reduce the flow of exciting impulses from the central nervous system that spill over into the sympathetic nervous system, constricting the arterioles and elevating pressure.

In addition to its work in the central nervous system,

reserpine acts in the sympathetic system, but not in the ganglia.

Remember those nerve fibers coming out of the ganglia and extending to the arterioles. Actually, the fibers stop just short of making contact with the receptors, or impulse-receiving sites, in the walls of the arterioles.

What happens is that when a nervous impulse traveling along a sympathetic nerve fiber reaches the end of the fiber, it causes the release of the chemical norepinephrine, which is actually made and stored in the fiber ending and differs from the chemical messenger at the synapse. It is the chemical that carries the message to the muscle fibers in the walls of arterioles, causing them to contract.

Reserpine (not to be confused with a blocking agent) acts to reduce the supply of norepinephrine in nerve endings and, by so doing, reduces the number of constricting impulses to the arterioles.

Like hydralazine, reserpine could sometimes produce side effects, especially with higher doses, most commonly, lethargy and mental depression.

But, with the development of reserpine and hydralazine, doctors had available two agents, effective by mouth, which could be used in treating moderate and mild hypertension. And, when combined, the two were cumulative or additive: smaller doses of each could be used, minimizing the likelihood of side effects.

THE USURPERS

A more recent drug is guanethidine, which, like reserpine, depletes the supply of norepinephrine in the nerve endings. But guanethidine goes a step further. It actually occupies the sites usually filled by norepinephrine.

As a result, guanethidine has a longer effect, remaining active for 10 to 14 days, often allowing smoother regulation of pressure. And, because its action is at the nerve endings and not on higher centers of the nervous system, it does not cause sedation or lethargy.

Another recently developed drug is methyldopa. It is related to a substance that the body employs in manufacturing norepinephrine, and the resemblance is great enough so that methyldopa can "worm" its way into the norepinephrine factory as a seemingly valuable raw material. But what is produced when methyldopa is used is alpha methyl norepinephrine rather than norepinephrine. And this altered form of norepinephrine, when released by a nervous impulse, is not as effective in passing along the signal to constrict the arteriole.

THE DIURETICS

Late in the 1950s, a new class of agents destined to become fundamental to the management of hypertension was discovered.

These are the thiazides—drugs derived from the sulfa compounds often used to combat bacterial infections. But instead of being infection fighters, thiazides are diuretics. They increase the kidneys' excretion of sodium and reduce fluid retention. The drugs, chlorothiazide and others, are effective when taken by mouth.

Investigators soon were discovering that chlorothiazide was as effective as severely restricted low salt diets in combating hypertension, and sometimes even more so.

Moreover, studies soon established that, in addition to lowering blood pressure on its own, chlorothiazide increased the response to other antihypertensive drugs. Often, only very small doses of other drugs had to be combined with chlorothiazide to produce excellent pressure reductions.

Finally, with the use of chlorothiazide or another diuretic of the same family, either alone or in combination with small amounts of other antihypertensives, it was possible to control blood pressure in most patients with little discomfort or inconvenience.

In just a few years, the drug treatment of hypertension had moved from cumbersome methods useful only for people with the most severe pressure elevations to a choice of agents, which, alone or in combination, were practical for all forms of hypertension.

Side effects still had to be considered. No drug, not even such a long and widely used one as aspirin, is effective and entirely safe for everybody. For that matter, not even any food is. Some people have idiosyncrasies that cause them to have unpleasant reactions to certain foods—anything from milk to shellfish—enjoyed by many millions of others.

But, with a choice of effective drugs, it had become possible to find one, or a combination of two or more, that could be effective for a particular patient with hypertension *with minimal or no side reactions.*

In addition to the drugs already mentioned, many others have been developed. Some have proved to be somewhat less effective than those mentioned. Others are under study. Some, already in wide use in Europe and elsewhere, have not yet passed through enough trials to permit them to be released for use in this country. Still others, very new ones, are in the early stages of investigation and may become available at some later date.

At present, the five antihypertensive agents available in the United States that have clearly established value and have passed the test of widespread use and the test of time as well are the thiazide diuretics, reserpine, hydralazine, guanethidine, and alpha-methyldopa.

THE RESULTS

The value of modern drug treatment has been dramatically demonstrated not only against one of the most severe forms of hypertension—malignant hypertension; survival has been greatly increased in other types of severe hypertension through reduction of deaths from complications. As blood pressure has been reduced, enlarged hearts have returned to normal size, signs and symptoms of heart failure have improved or even disappeared entirely, kidney deterioration has been arrested, the threat of strokes has diminished.

It remained for the Veterans Administration study, by

Dr. Edward Freis and his colleagues in 17 VA hospitals across the country, to provide a dramatic demonstration of the value of modern drug therapy in mild and moderate hypertension. The results—first among patients with diastolic pressures ranging from 115 to 129, the moderate hypertensives, some of whom received drug treatment while others, for comparison, did not—could hardly be ignored. Over an extended period, there were no deaths and only one nonfatal stroke and one nonfatal heart attack among those receiving treatment, contrasted with 4 deaths and 27 serious heart attacks and strokes among the others.

Nor could there have been a much more impressive demonstration of the value of treating mild hypertension than the second VA study covering patients with blood pressures of 90 to 114. Compared with other patients with such pressures not receiving treatment, those who were put on drug treatment showed a two-thirds reduction in the risk of developing stroke or heart attack and whereas a sizable proportion of the untreated patients went on to progress from mild hypertension to severe hypertension, none of the treated patients did.

Today, with such results to go on, more and more physicians are convinced that there is a great opportunity, through early detection and treatment of milder degrees of hypertension, to prevent progression of the disease. New campaigns by local and national agencies or groups, covered in the Appendix, reflect this evaluation.

9

Arriving at the Right Treatment for You

When his blood pressure turned out to be elevated on first measurement, there was no rush to treat him for it. The first reading for George was 155/102.

In anyone—more so in an anxious individual but in others as well—the mere act of having a blood pressure measurement has a pressor effect. It tends to increase the pressure.

The measurement was repeated later in the visit. The pressure remained elevated. It was still elevated a week later when George returned, at the physician's request, to have his blood pressure taken by the office nurse. And that was true still another week later.

Meanwhile, the physician had delved thoroughly into George's family history. Did either of his parents or any of his sisters or brothers have hypertension? Had they had any complications of hypertension? If any had died, what had caused death and at what age had it occurred?

In George's case, his father had died at a relatively early age of a heart attack. An older brother had been having some trouble with angina chest pains. It does not require a long family history of hypertension and serious consequences to establish that blood pressure elevation is going to be a significant problem for an individual. There can be serious consequences of uncontrolled hypertension without such a history. But such a familial pattern definitely suggests that the chances of trouble will be great.

119

If George's family had been free of hypertension, that very fact could serve to alert the doctor to the possibility of some possibly curable form of hypertension. Even with a definite family history of hypertension, such a possibility cannot be dismissed offhand; the lack of family history is simply one clue.

Many tests are available to check for the various relatively rare but curable forms of hypertension. In George's case, his physician compared leg blood pressure measurements with those in an arm, found them much the same, and could rule out coarctation of the aorta. His chest X ray showed no notching of the ribs, another rule-out of coarctation. His very appearance indicated he did not have Cushing's syndrome. Urine and blood tests quickly removed any suspicion of adrenal gland tumor or urinary tract infection.

An electrocardiogram showed that George had only a slight enlargement of the left ventricle of the heart as a result of hypertension. His physician checked his eyes with an ophthalmoscope, an instrument capable of making visible any damage caused by hypertension to the small vessels— the arterioles—in the retina.

All the indications were that George had essential hypertension, not related to any operable underlying cause, that, fortunately, had been detected early; as yet there were no serious complications.

THERE IS NO ONE SET—AND BEST— PROCEDURE FOR ESTABLISHING THE DIAGNOSIS OF HYPERTENSION AND THE NEED FOR TREATMENT

For one thing, each physician may have some variations of his own, some procedures that, in his experience, he finds generally most helpful.

Patients vary too. They vary in age, in family history, in reactions to medical examinations, and in still other respects. It's often necessary to vary the procedures according to the individual patient.

Even in the matter of just determining whether hypertension actually exists, for example, a few blood pressure measurements may be enough. At the other extreme, however, for some patients some physicians find it advisable to give a family member a manometer (sphygmomanometer). They teach him its use and have him take the measurements repeatedly over a period of several days or weeks—to make certain that the elevations are true elevations requiring treatment rather than temporary excessive responses to apprehension in the physician's office.

THE AIM OF TREATMENT

Once it is established that the hypertension is real and persistent, and that, as is true in the vast majority of cases, it is essential hypertension without an underlying possibly curable cause, the approach to treatment, as with diagnosis, may vary considerably from patient to patient.

The aim of treatment is to bring down the blood pressure to normal or near-normal levels and keep it there. It is also to accomplish this with minimal side effects or—and this is increasingly possible—without side effects at all.

The ideal treatment program is not only one that can turn a hypertensive patient into a normotensive individual, but also treatment with which he can live comfortably.

If it is to be comfortable, it has to be suited to the individual patient.

Commonly it requires drugs, selected drugs. Sometimes, it requires no drugs at all.

Before considering drug treatment, if you are overweight, your physician may suggest a trial period of reducing. If the hypertension is quite mild, weight reduction sometimes may be all that is needed to reestablish normal blood pressure. Successful weight reduction, as indicated in Chapter 7, may not be an easy matter, but it can be accomplished if approached intelligently; it has much to recommend it in addition to its usefulness in controlling elevated blood pressure.

Similarly, if your salt intake happens to be high (Chapter 7), your physician may suggest some moderation.

There may be suggestions, too, if they seem pertinent in your case, on exercise and how you might perhaps handle stressful situations more effectively (Chapter 7).

Whatever the physician's recommendations, he will want to see you within a specified time to check on results.

DRUGS

When drugs are needed, the choice is highly selective.

Many physicians often find it advisable to begin with a thiazide diuretic. Through its effect on the excretion of salt and excess fluid (Chapter 8), such an agent may bring pressure down to normal levels. It may be used in smaller doses twice a day or in a larger dose once a day. Within a few weeks to a month, it should be clear whether a diuretic alone will suffice.

If the blood pressure falls to normal levels with a diuretic, your physician may then try a smaller dose, seeking to establish the minimum necessary to keep your blood pressure down.

A word of caution: though diuretic treatment has obviated the need for a stringent low-salt diet, consuming very large amounts of salt (25 grams a day, which is well in excess of the average 15 grams a day) can nullify a thiazide's antihypertensive effect; excretion can't keep up with intake.

Oral thiazide diuretics are probably the most widely used of all antihypertensive agents. Some thiazides are effective for short periods, some longer, even 24 hours. No one diuretic has a singular advantage. Especially in mild hypertension, an oral diuretic may be effective in itself.

When a diuretic alone does not suffice, one of the other drugs may be added. Many physicians find reserpine an excellent drug for its effectiveness in combination with a diuretic, its convenience of use, and low cost. It does not, of course, work for all patients. In some, even if effective, it may not be advisable since, unlike for many others, it may have mentally depressive effects or produce gastrointestinal upsets.

In small doses hydralazine is often effective for patients

who fail to respond adequately to thiazide alone. Hydralazine often is effective, too, for patients who do not respond adequately to a combination of thiazide and reserpine.

Whereas alpha-methyldopa usually is employed in combination with a diuretic, it alone can achieve a long-term blood pressure reduction for a small number of patients.

In the experience of many physicians in private practice and research, with one or another program of drug treatment—diuretic alone, diuretic plus reserpine, diuretic plus hydralazine, diuretic plus methyldopa, or methyldopa alone —more than 90 percent of essential hypertension patients can achieve effective control.

Guanethidine is usually reserved for treating severe hypertension. It is a potent drug, not simple to use; the dosage must be carefully fitted to the patient; but it can be effective when other agents are not fully satisfactory in bringing down severe elevations of pressure.

Some patients with severe hypertension who do not respond adequately to other drugs respond well to a diuretic plus clonidine—a drug similar to methyldopa.

Spironolactone, an aldosterone-blocking agent, with a pressure-lowering effect, may be used for patients with primary aldosteronism (Chapter 6). Sometimes, when in a few patients long-continued thiazide diuretic treatment ceases to produce the necessary response, spironolactone can effect substantial blood-pressure reduction. Spironolactone also may be added to treatment under other special circumstances, such as for patients who also have gout.

ONCE-A-DAY TREATMENT

Modern treatment for hypertension to some extent may even be tailored to the personality of the patient.

Some people don't mind—and may even brag of—following elaborate drug programs. Others resent frequent pill taking.

Even when several drugs must be used, based on minimum needs, there need not be any complicated ritual.

Moreover, in many cases a pill a day will suffice. At

least 50 percent of all mild to moderate hypertension patients respond just to a thiazide diuretic and we have already
seen that some of the longer-acting thiazides need be taken
only once a day.

Also, drug combinations of various kinds are available in
single-tablet form. Frequently combinations, thiazide and
reserpine for example, are suitable after a patient's blood
pressure has been brought down to normal; one tablet a day
may provide adequate maintenance.

HOME MEASUREMENTS

For some patients, taking blood pressure measurements at
home may be of value.

Not all physicians agree that this is ever really essential.
What bothers them is the possibility of patient overconcern,
of inducing a blood-pressure neurosis. But it all depends on
the individuality of the patient. Some physicians report that
when patients record blood pressures at home regularly,
over long periods, the procedure becomes routine and usually loses any capacity for producing anxiety.

Home measurements may help to assure proper treatment
not only in patients who tend to be overreactors during office
measurements but in others as well. Once a treatment program has been established, twice-a-day recordings at home
(most conveniently, in many cases, in the morning on arising
and at bedtime), with the readings noted and submitted
perhaps once a month to the physician, may reduce office
visits to once or twice a year and yet allow proper assessment
of the adequacy of treatment.

Other physicians find home blood-pressure readings have
another value for some patients—motivation. Patients can
see for themselves that regularly taken medications are having an effect.

Measuring blood pressure is a simple enough procedure
and most people can learn it readily in a short time with a
little instruction from a physician or a physician's assistant.

Wrap the cuff of the instrument around your upper left

arm. Then, after placing the stethoscope earpieces in your ears, pump the hand bulb with your left hand.

Next, bending the left arm a bit, use your right hand to place the cone-shaped end of the stethoscope over the artery at the elbow. Now, you pump the hand bulb some more until the expanding cuff has stopped the pulse in the artery (you will recognize this when you no longer hear any beats through the stethoscope).

Next, you let air slowly escape from the bulb by twisting the valve on it. As you let out the air slowly, you listen for beating sounds to come through the stethoscope. As soon as you begin to hear these beats, you read the number on the mercury column showing the height of the mercury. This number indicates the systolic blood pressure, the higher value, when the heart beats.

Now, as you let more air escape from the bulb, you will reach a point where the beats begin to fade away. At this point, the level of mercury in the column will show—even though the sounds have not completely disappeared but only begun to fade away—the diastolic or lower pressure measuring in-between beats of the heart.

New manometers, specially designed for use by patients, may make home measurements even more simple.

However, the value of taking home blood-pressure measurements should be decided in consultation with a physician. It is certainly no absolute requirement for proper treatment.

OVERCOMING ANY SIDE EFFECTS

As with foods, pollens, aspirin, and many other drugs, antihypertensive agents produce varying reactions depending on the individual. The physician must determine which drug or drugs may be most effective, while avoiding undesirable side effects. Treatment must be well tolerated.

You may be fortunate, as many people are, in that an effective, well-tolerated program to control your blood pressure is arrived at quickly, perhaps even at once. If some experimentation is in order, however, it is well worthwhile. It may include adjustment of dosage or change in drugs used so as to eliminate undesirable effects. Obviously, any side effects should be reported promptly to your physician for correction.

DIURETIC SIDE EFFECTS

Since diuretic drugs remove salt from the body, it might be expected that they remove other chemicals. In particular, in some patients, they may remove too much potassium. If only a bit too much potassium is removed, there is seldom any trouble. If a considerable amount is removed, muscle weakness may follow. The answer often is simply to put back the lost potassium by drinking citrus juices, for example, several glasses of orange juice daily, or by increasing the intake of foods rich in potassium, as suggested by the physician.

Particularly for patients who are also receiving the heart drug digitalis, potassium loss may make the digitalis more likely to produce abnormal heart rhythms. For them, a potassium-sparing diuretic (such as spironolactone or triamterene) may be used in addition to the thiazide diuretic. If there is a satisfactory response, a capsule containing the combination may be used thereafter.

Thiazide diuretics also may sometimes precipitate gout in patients with a history of the disorder. But its likelihood can be minimized by drugs commonly used to help prevent gout attacks (probenecid or allopurinol).

RESERPINE SIDE EFFECTS

The most important side effect of reserpine is severe mental depression. This is far from inevitable. When it occurs, it most likely afflicts patients with histories of depressive illness. Some of the symptoms of depression may include anxiety, despondency, unaccustomed early rising, and loss of appetite. If depression does develop, it almost invariably disappears within a few days after the drug is discontinued; any depressive reactions to it should be reported immediately to the physician to save unnecessary suffering. Sometimes, once the depressive effects are gone, reserpine may be used successfully in smaller doses, or the patient can be switched readily to other antihypertensive medication.

Some patients experience a sensation of lethargy from reserpine treatment, but a decline in ambition or pep should not be confused with depression; patients experiencing lethargy do not wake early in the morning as do those experiencing depression, nor do they lose their appetites. Actually, some patients welcome their lethargy. They become less uptight and may enjoy life more. But lethargy does not have to become a problem for any patient: a decrease in reserpine dosage may eliminate the side effects or, if necessary, a switch can be made to another antihypertensive agent.

Nasal stuffiness and slight diarrhea are other possible side effects. The problem of a stuffy nose may be so slight as to produce little discomfort; on the other hand, some patients have a "cold" as long as they take reserpine and it is sometimes necessary to stop the drug for a week until the cold symptom clears.

Another possible side effect is after-midnight dreaming, which may disturb sleep. There are no nightmares but, rather, bizarre dreams, that are not necessarily unpleasant. If the reserpine is discontinued for a week, the dreams often stop, and thereafter lesser doses of reserpine may not produce them and yet still produce a good pressure-lowering effect.

HYDRALAZINE SIDE EFFECTS

In some patients, hydralazine may produce headaches. In a few cases, the headaches may be continuous and incapacitating as long as the drug is used, and so another drug may have to be used in its place. But far more often, if headaches occur at all, they disappear spontaneously as treatment continues. Any headaches at the start of hydralazine therapy should be reported to the physician, but there may be no need to immediately discontinue the drug.

Sometimes hydralazine may produce such side effects as weakness, palpitation, nausea, and, occasionally, chest pain of the angina type. Such side effects were more common when hydralazine was used in larger doses as the sole treatment; they are much less frequent now that smaller doses, in combination with other medication, are employed. But when any such side effects give persistent trouble, they do not have to be tolerated. If still smaller doses of hydralazine avoid the problems and still control the blood pressure, the drug may be continued. Otherwise, another drug may be used.

Sometimes, in large doses—greater than 200 milligrams a day—hydralazine may produce arthritis-like symptoms and skin eruptions, and these may require a modification of treatment.

ALPHA-METHYLDOPA SIDE EFFECTS

A small proportion of patients cannot take effective doses of methyldopa because the drug makes them excessively sleepy. For some, dryness of the mouth may be an undesirable effect. One broadcasting personality, with his hypertension well enough controlled with methyldopa, couldn't continue on the drug because his mouth became so dry he couldn't function effectively on the job. He could switch readily enough to another agent.

Occasionally, some patients experience postural hypotension—postural low blood pressure. In such cases, there is enough of a reduction in blood pressure when the person assumes an erect position to make him feel temporarily faint, especially when he assumes that position suddenly.

One relatively uncommon major side effect in some patients is hepatitis, or liver inflammation, which is generally mild. It usually occurs within the first six weeks of treatment and is manifested by fever and malaise or general discomfort. Recovery is rapid when the drug is discontinued.

GUANETHIDINE SIDE EFFECTS

Guanethidine is an extremely potent drug, valuable in severe hypertension, also useful for milder hypertension. But for some people it may bring burdensome side effects.

It is more likely than other drugs to produce postural hypotension and faintness. When it does, the drug may not have to be discontinued; careful adjustment of dosage may bring excellent control of pressure with minimal trouble from postural hypotension.

Diarrhea sometimes is another troublesome side effect. It usually does not disappear unless the dose is reduced, sometimes to an ineffective level. But certain other drugs, called anticholinergic agents, which have no effect on blood pressure, often can control the diarrhea, permitting continued use of guanethidine.

Guanethidine sometimes may affect sexual function in men, yet most men on the drug do not object too much. They can have erections but ejaculation is backward—into the urinary bladder—so there is no emission. Except for that, sexual function is fairly normal.

A TRUE PICTURE

Listing the side effects may make antihypertensive drugs sound formidable. But that is not the case.

As we have noted previously, no food, no beverage, no drug is "kind" to every person. Some people simply do not tolerate foods that others find innocuous and delicious. Milk, a highly desirable food for babies, is intolerable to some. Coffee, a habit for many, is for some a cause of jitters or worse. Alcohol, perhaps the world's oldest and most widely used "tranquilizer" and "relaxant," acts as a stimulant in some people, producing bizarre effects.

Antibiotic drugs have saved millions of lives, but they have had some undesirable effects, too, leading to the development of new infections while curing original ones. Cortisone and similar agents have proved extremely valuable, often lifesaving, for people with ailments ranging from severe allergies and asthma to arthritis and severe kidney diseases, but they have produced their share of undesirable effects, even including mental upsets.

For most people, antihypertensive drugs are effective. For most people, there are no undesirable reactions to most of the drugs. And, for virtually all hypertensives, the right drug or combination of drugs in the right dosage can be found so that blood pressure can be controlled with minimal or no discomfort at all.

Knowing about possible side effects of antihypertensive agents does not necessarily mean that you will ever experience them. If you should experience them, you will have some understanding of their significance. You will be aware of their connection with treatment and be able to call them to the attention of your physician. If you do that, you can be virtually certain that the side effects will be minimized or eliminated entirely through a modification or change of treatment that still provides effective control of your blood pressure.

10

Living the Full Life

She was only 34 years old when the crisis struck. She had a blood pressure reading of 260/140. Her heart was enlarged; her neck veins distended; her ankles swollen with fluid. She was unable to lie flat in bed or even walk to the bathroom because of shortness of breath. For a month, too, she had had recurring episodes of blood spitting.

She was hospitalized and it took a combination of three drugs to bring her blood pressure down. She also had to have digitalis to buck up her laboring, overburdened heart. She lost 60 pounds in 4 weeks, most of it excess fluid. Her heart size began to decrease, and her shortness of breath to disappear. She is now still on antihypertensive medication, but free of marked disability; she does her household work, shops, and can walk up several flights of stairs.

Six years ago, at the age of 43, he suffered a crippling stroke when an artery in his brain, long weakened by excessive blood pressure, ballooned and burst. His right side, arm, and leg were paralyzed.

His high blood pressure had been discovered first, many years before, when he failed an army physical examination. But that was before there was effective drug control for hypertension. He didn't worry about his pressure. He felt fine for years. But then came the stroke.

He is a well-known writer and he has told his story succinctly. "Rehabilitation restored my limbs to normal motion and, while I was in the hospital, my doctors worked out the most effective combination of drugs to hold my blood pressure, which had shot all the way up to 220/140, to normal levels. For six months after I left the hospital, my doctor checked me once a month. Now I visit him only two or three times a year. I agree with my doctor when he tells me: 'Your treatment isn't successful if it interferes with your normal life. You can't stop living.' And I haven't." He is normally active, if anything even more so than before; he travels extensively, writes prolifically, enjoys life.

Even after complications have begun, control of hypertension can have great value. It can't erase all the complications, such as damage to artery walls, but it may markedly reduce such damage as the enlargement of the heart and pumping weakness. It has great potential for extending life. That has been shown clearly in many studies in which, when patients with severe hypertension and advanced complications were aggressively treated to normalize their blood pressure, their mortality rates over a period of years were reduced by as much as two-thirds in comparison with others not so treated.

Control of hypertension before complications occur has even greater potential.

Even a little high blood pressure, one authority has remarked, is "like a little pregnancy—you have trouble."

Life insurance studies have clearly shown that a blood pressure of around 100/60 is associated with the longest life expectancy. With levels of pressure from 120/80 to 140/90 —still within the "normal range"—the mortality rate rises a bit. When blood pressure is definitely in the hypertensive range, life expectancy is reduced still further.

Effective, practical drug treatment for hypertension is a recent development. As is often the case with medical advances, the first large-scale applications of antihypertensive drug treatment involved patients with moderate and severe blood pressure elevations.

And the treatment has proved valuable in many ways. It didn't matter whether a patient was 15, 25, 40, 50, or well beyond 70 years old. Used consistently, the treatment brought down blood pressures, reduced morbidity and sickness, and helped prevent many deadly events.

There has *not* been a complete elimination of *all* deadly events, but there has been a marked reduction in *many*.

The fact is that the most striking gains in patients with moderate and severe elevations given effective antihypertensive drug treatment have been in the prevention of strokes and congestive heart failure. There is still room for further improvement in these areas, and it is almost certain to come as drug treatment now is applied increasingly to milder elevations so that the moderate and severe elevations are avoided, further minimizing the risk of complications by giving them less opportunity to develop.

And it's in such early treatment for mild elevations that the big hope for preventing advanced coronary heart disease and heart attacks lies.

Coronary heart disease can be looked upon, in a way, as a kind of special case of atherosclerosis.

Though atherosclerosis, with its buildup of clogging fat deposits, can affect virtually any artery in the body, it has a special predilection for the coronary arteries. Nobody knows precisely why, but it can begin its encroachment there earlier and advance more intensively than in other arteries.

With the evidence now that hypertension may play a double role in coronary atherosclerosis—producing structural changes in the inner artery walls that may make the walls more susceptible to deposits and then possibly pounding in the deposits—the need is to control hypertension early, the earlier the better in terms of reducing the opportunity for atherosclerosis to get started or, if it has started, to advance very far.

And it now appears that we are entering an era in which a cardinal aim of medicine will be not only to treat hypertension any time it is found but to be alert for it, find it early, and treat it as early as possible.

SOME REALITIES

It could be an era marking one of the most important advances ever made in preventive medicine.

Certainly other factors in heart and blood vessel disease deserve attention: the fats in our diet and the fats in our

blood, excessive smoking, modes of life virtually devoid of
physical effort, and still others.

But of all factors, hypertension ranks not only as one of
critical importance but also as the one that is most amenable—immediately—to practical control.

Yet, one fact must be faced. The control of hypertension
does not lie entirely with the physician. It lies primarily
with the patient.

In an essay called "Patient, Heal Thyself," Dr. Eric R.
Sanderson recently wrote:

"You may remember the story of the man who bought the
mule. The seller assured him that if the mule stopped he
would go again if the buyer spoke in his ear, 'Giddy-up. Get
going.' So the mule stopped and the man said, 'Giddy-up.
Get going,' and nothing happened. The man sought out the
seller and told him what had transpired. The seller picked
up a large two-by-four, walked over to the mule and struck
him squarely between the eyes. Then he said to the mule,
'Giddy-up. Get going,' and the mule did. 'See,' the seller
said. 'He'll do what you tell him to do, but first you have
to get his attention.'"

Yet, as Dr. Sanderson went on to note, even after people
are made aware of problems and consequences, "it is very
difficult to get them to do anything. . . . Most people do
not like to assume responsibility for their own fate. They are
inclined to slough it off and let somebody else take the blame
when things go wrong."

If this is true for matters of health, it is especially so for
hypertension and its control.

One big problem is to get the patient to the physician
when he is feeling well—for a checkup to see whether or not
his blood pressure is elevated.

Another problem is to get the patient to continue treatment when he is feeling well.

It's nothing new that many patients fail to follow physician's orders. Studies at the University of Southern California indicate that overall, for all types of health problems,
up to 35 percent, or more, of the patients ignore or com-
promise medical advice and instructions. In some cases, it is

because patients deny illness; they don't like to think of themselves as having a problem. In some cases, they don't like restrictions such as bed rest and reduced work; they see these as threats to their way of life. In some cases, after seeing a doctor, they go home and become diverted by the well-meant but usually uninformed and useless advice of a relative or friend. In some cases, they blame expense or inconvenience of treatment.

But the "dropout" problem—the failure to continue treatment—can become particularly acute when the patient has no symptoms. And we've seen that hypertension does not necessarily produce symptoms; in fact, symptoms are very rare for mild or even moderate hypertension. Most often, the symptoms come when the hypertension has been long active and has already produced complications.

As noted earlier, it is estimated that half of all the 24 million or more hypertensives in the United States are undetected. They have no symptoms, so do not get a medical checkup. Half of those who are detected and know they are hypertensive and go untreated do so because they have no symptoms.

Failing to recognize or to thoroughly appreciate that hypertension is "the silent killer" and that lack of symptoms means nothing, they shrug off treatment.

Is it bother to keep blood pressure under control? At first there may be considerable bother, until treatment is precisely adjusted to individual need. But, thereafter, there is usually less and less bother, and the control of hypertension becomes routine, a matter of course, part of the way of life.

FREEDOM TO LIVE WELL

After satisfying himself about your overall condition, about the condition of your heart and blood vessels, your physician will have advice about what you can and cannot do.

There is a good likelihood that you will not only be able to work as you always have; you may be able to work more efficiently. There is a good likelihood that you will be able to play, to enjoy recreation, to participate in sports, to be fully active, and you may even be encouraged to be more active as an additional way of increasing your prospects for longer, healthier life.

"Unnecessary restrictions on normal living habits should be avoided," says Dr. Edward Freis. "There is no point in imposing a rigidly restricted low-sodium diet if thiazides are being given. There is no reason to restrict moderate exercise within the limits of the patient's competence. Alcohol taken in moderation is beneficial."

Sir George Pickering, one of the great names in high blood pressure research and treatment and a world authority, expresses a conviction many physicians share: "A cardinal rule is to avoid petty interference with liberty and the enjoyment of life. Patients with elevated arterial pressure should not be allowed to become fat, otherwise restrictions should only be imposed because of the presence of complications and not from fear of them."

Note that significant last point: ". . . not from fear of them."

Hypertension may stem from any of many causes, perhaps including some still unknown. And if a cause can be found which is curable, fine.

But the danger of hypertension is not in the cause. Rather, it lies in the blood pressure elevation itself.

"Regardless of cause, the morbid complications of hypertension," observes Dr. Edward N. Ehrlich of the Department of Medicine, University of Chicago, "are consequences of the blood pressure elevations themselves."

Reducing the pressure, even if the cause remains, is what counts. It is bringing the pressure down toward normal that can help to prevent the complications.

And, thus, as Sir George Pickering observes, when a patient with hypertension is treated and has no complications, which is all the more likely if the pressure elevation is found and treated early, then restrictions on living do not have to be imposed because of fear that this or that activity will bring on complications. Given proper treatment, carried out faithfully by the patient, Pickering maintains there is no need to be afraid that complications will ensue.

The writer mentioned earlier, whose hypertension, far advanced, had led to a paralyzing stroke, observed: "The outlook for me, as for the multitude of persons hit by high blood pressure sometime during life, has never been brighter. Though I am not cured, my disease *is* being managed. Since my stroke, I have traveled more than a quarter of a million miles to more than 40 countries, even passed the four-hour-long physical examination given to Royal Swedish Air Force pilots annually. I have been a war correspondent in Vietnam, and last June I celebrated my 50th birthday by climbing an Austrian Alp."

His physician had told him: "Your treatment isn't successful if it interferes with your normal life. You can't stop living." He hasn't.

Nor need you.

Hypertension is a killer that now can be tamed. And if you have it, its taming can give you the freedom to live a longer, healthier life.

11

Coming Events

MARIJUANA

Recently, at McGill University in Montreal, researchers were carrying out studies, in animals, with the main active ingredient in marijuana, delta-9-THC, when they found that it produced significant reductions in blood pressure.

Within an hour after they injected a moderate dose of the THC compound into rats with experimentally induced hypertension, the blood pressure levels dropped and remained at lowered levels for several hours. There were no overt behavioral or bodily side effects. After a week of treatment, the blood pressures of treated rats were significantly lower than those of untreated ones.

In another test, rats bred to be hypertensive—with blood pressure elevations believed to be similar to those common in human hypertensive patients—were injected with a crude extract of marijuana. Again blood pressure levels were lowered.

Marijuana or its THC ingredient may or may not have any practical significance as a means of controlling elevated blood pressure. But the McGill work is only one example of the continuing, and growing, hypertension research effort.

Whole new classes of drugs are being investigated. So are potentially useful drugless treatments.

ELECTRONIC STIMULATION

In rare cases essential hypertension may fail to respond to any drug treatment or combination of drug treatments. The reason for the failure is not clear.

But even for these, promising results are being obtained with a small electronic device implanted in the neck region so as to stimulate the nerves in the carotid sinus—a center involved in the body's control of blood pressure. Power for the device is beamed from an external battery pack and transmitter.

Physicians at Philadelphia's Hahnemann Medical College have used the device successfully in a series of patients with otherwise unyielding hypertension. Blood pressure that had been running as high as 240/150 and even higher fell to near-normal levels within a short time after the electronic device was put to use.

A DIRECT APPROACH

A direct approach could involve using drugs that can dilate arterioles. But such drugs, called vasodilators, have also tended to stimulate the heart.

However, a new vasodilator (minoxidil) is now available for study, and it appears to have greater dilating power than previous ones. Also, another drug, propranolol, can counterbalance any heart stimulation. In studies thus far the combination of the two agents, with a diuretic added, appears promising. Markedly elevated blood pressures in human patients have been brought down to normal or near-normal levels. Side effects apparently are no problem and an additional advantage of minoxidil may be its prolonged activity; it is showing continuing effectiveness over a period of several days.

THE NEWEST HORMONES

Much fascinated scientific attention today is focused on the possibilities that may lie in a striking new class of compounds, natural body hormones unknown until very recently.

The compounds, called prostaglandins, are under study in more than 500 laboratories around the world. New scientific reports on them have been appearing at a rate of two a day.

Those reports indicate that prostaglandins, if they live up to their promise, may provide a whole shelfful of highly effective medicines.

Some prostaglandins appear to be capable of opening closed airways to the lungs, indicating potential usefulness in treating asthma and emphysema. Some clear clogged nasal passages familiar to common cold sufferers. There are prostaglandins that shut off the secretion of stomach acid, suggesting possible value for peptic ulcer control. Some can induce labor in pregnant women. Some, used in the early weeks of pregnancy, can produce therapeutic abortions. At least one of the prostaglandins appears to hold promise as a once-a-month contraception suppository, and there are trials of the drugs for improving male fertility and for the treatment of arthritis.

The prostaglandins also are showing promise in lowering blood pressure, apparently without undesirable side effects.

The compounds—thus far 14 have been identified and there may be others—are present in humans and all other mammals. They are classified as hormones. But whereas the well-known hormones produced by the thyroid, pituitary, adrenals, and other glands circulate through the body in the blood and act on distant target organs, the prostaglandins are produced by virtually every tissue of the body and act locally, on the spot. They are involved in normal body functioning; they are also sometimes involved in disease.

The first clue to the existence of the compounds was in 1930, but apparently it was forgotten. Two New York City gynecologists, interested in problems of fertility and sterility, at that time discovered that strips of uterine tissue from women with histories of successful pregnancies relaxed when exposed to fresh male semen but tissue from sterile women contracted instead. If the two men followed up that lead at all, they did not report on it.

Then, three years later, investigators in England and Sweden, working independently, found that when they injected into test animals either human semen or extracts of sheep vesicular glands, which produce semen, smooth muscle contracted and blood pressure was lowered. Neither effect could be accounted for by any known agents in the semen or gland extracts. The name prostaglandin—suggesting prostate-gland origin for the mysterious material, was coined by Professor Ulf S. von Euler, who later was to win a Nobel Prize for other work. The name has stuck, although prostaglandins since have been found produced in many other places in the body.

It was not until 1957 that two different prostaglandins were actually isolated. It took another five years to establish their chemical architecture. By 1968, however, not only had other prostaglandins been isolated, but one after another of them began to be synthesized, produced artificially in the laboratory. And since then it has become possible, because of the increased supply of the materials, to begin to do intensive research on the functions and potential values of the fourteen known prostaglandins.

Actually, almost 25 years ago, a German researcher had discovered a substance produced by the intestines that influenced bowel contractions; he named it darmstoff. Ten years later, a Welsh physiologist found a substance that produced powerful contractions of the uterus during menstruation and called it "menstrual stimulant." In 1965, Dr. James B. Lee and a St. Louis University team found something in the rabbit kidney that could lower blood pressure. Now all three substances have been shown to be prostaglandins.

It now appears that the long-mystifying mechanism of action for aspirin may lie in the fact that aspirin counters the activities of a prostaglandin that, under some circumstances, produces fever, headaches, and inflammation.

Some researchers believe that prostaglandins are part of a vast monitoring system of the body, and that they may encourage or inhibit the activities of the better-known hormones. The fascinating mechanism may be this: the better-known hormones are really messengers transmitting messages that are to be carried out within body cells. The carrying out is the responsibility of a remarkable substance called cyclic AMP, a versatile "second messenger." But a critical factor for the production of cyclic AMP is an enzyme in the cell wall. Prostaglandins may control this enzyme and thus control cyclic AMP production and the ability of the cell to carry out hormonal instructions. Put another way, prostaglandins appear to be the only known agents capable of raising the level of cyclic AMP in some cells and decreasing it in others.

Dr. Lee believes that a deficiency of certain prostaglandins naturally present in the kidneys may explain many if not most cases of hypertension. Actually, more than a decade ago, while at Harvard, Dr. Lee found that kidney extracts injected into test animals produced a marked blood pressure drop. He has since found that three active compounds in kidney tissue are three different prostaglandins. It appears that the sole job of one of them is to lower blood pressure. Animal experiments suggest that it does so by relaxing small blood vessels, thus easing blood flow.

Dr. Lee, who now is studying prostaglandins in human hypertensive patients, has succeeded in reducing pressures from a mean elevation of 200/100 to 140/80. He has also noted that blood flow to the kidneys is increased and the excretion of salt and water is also increased—both desirable reactions.

The prostaglandins are still considered experimental drugs. Much more research will be needed before they become available for everyday medical use. But the pace of that research is very rapid.

MIND CONTROL

Perhaps hypertensive patients ultimately will control their blood pressures mentally, obviating the need for drugs or other measures.

Investigators in many laboratories have been finding that

blood pressures in animals can be made to rise and fall predictably; that squirrel monkeys with induced hypertension can be trained by conditioning techniques to lower their blood pressures; and that by similar procedures human subjects can be trained to raise and lower pressure.

For thousands of years, mystics and yogis have claimed remarkable control over mind and body, including the ability even to drop the pulse to the vanishing point. Westerners generally have scoffed at this. They have based their scoffing on the fact that there are two nervous systems—that, supposedly, while one, the voluntary nervous system, is under the control of the conscious mind, the other, the autonomic or involuntary system, is not—and it is this autonomic system which controls the activities of the heart, blood vessels, and visceral organs.

But now, through a technique called biofeedback, investigators have been able to show that the autonomic nervous system is not so autonomic after all; that man can learn to control his internal organs much as he does his arms, legs, and other body parts.

The principle behind biofeedback is basically simple. We learn to do many things by virtue of visual and neuromuscular feedback cues. For example, in playing tennis, we feel an arm move, see how the racquet connects with the ball, see where the ball goes, and the next time correct the arm movement.

Biofeedback cues can be obtained through laboratory instruments that pick up and amplify blood pressure changes and heart rate changes. The instruments are not new—only this application of them is. They are hooked up to produce sound or light signals, and the individual, through the signals, can get cues for internal changes.

When, for example, he sees a light indicating that his blood pressure has risen, then sees another indicating the pressure has fallen, he can begin to remember the internal sensation associated with each and then may learn to induce the sensation associated with the desired light.

Much of the pioneering work in biofeedback was done by psychologist Neal E. Miller and his colleagues at New

York's Rockefeller University. In many ingenious experiments, Miller by making use of rewards was able to get dogs to increase and decrease heart rate, intestinal contractions, and blood pressure. He reached the point of being able to train rats, in just 90 minutes, to increase or decrease their heart rates by an average of 20 percent. And when retested several months later, the animals still retained the ability to control heart rate.

Currently, at many institutions, diverse trials are under way with human volunteers, seriously exploring the potential of biofeedback to help in many health problems.

For example, migraine with its throbbing pain is believed to result from pressure in enlarged blood vessels in the head. Can patients learn to prevent the headaches through mental control? It seems so from studies at the Menninger Foundation in Topeka, Kansas.

At its clinic, migraine patients are seated in an easy chair in a quiet laboratory room. A temperature-sensing electrode is taped to a finger and another is taped to the forehead. On a table before them, they can see a meter that shows the difference between head temperature and hand temperaure.

They are asked to move the needle on the meter to the right, which requires that hand temperature be raised and that, in turn, requires relaxing blood vessels. The relaxation and the redistribution of blood flow that may accompany it apparently is of value in migraine. Once the patients develop some ability to move the needle and some sense of how they accomplish the moving, they find that, wherever they are, they can use the same technique to cut short a migraine attack.

In trials at Baltimore City Hospital, investigators are working with patients suffering from premature ventricular contraction, a potentially dangerous heartbeat irregularity. Through electrodes taped to the chest, heartbeats are made to trigger light. When a patient sees a green light, he knows he should try to speed his heart rate; a red light indicates he should try to slow the rate. After about ten sessions of more than an hour each, many patients are able to change heart rate on command—and also are able to do the same thing at home without instrumentation and thus control their symptoms.

At the Hypertension Clinic of the Boston City Hospital, similar techniques have been used for patients with high blood pressure. In one study, five men and two women learned to decrease their systolic pressures by as much as 33.8 points.

Studies are under way elsewhere as well—at Rockefeller University, Harvard Medical School, the Lafayette Clinic in Detroit—on teaching hypertensive patients to control blood pressure by biofeedback.

The work is promising but as yet not definitive. Can such control serve for prolonged periods out of the laboratory as well as in? Would it work for most if not all patients? Would it require some change in behavior and even of life-style as well as a period of biofeedback training? These are questions yet to be answered.

Many investigators believe that biofeedback has great promise for hypertension control.

They consider that elevated pressure is related to the continuous physical and behavioral adjustments that must be made in response to environmental conditions. The autonomic nervous system adjustments to the environment, evolved and stabilized thousands of years ago, involved a temporary increase in blood pressure to help mobilize body energy for fight or flight in response to alarming situations. It seems somewhat anachronistic now.

Dr. Herbert Benson of Harvard and Boston City Hospital notes: "This response, suitable previously, is now often inappropriate and may lead to permanent hypertension, especially since our environment has changed and is becoming more complex and unpredictable at an accelerating pace.

"Since the apparently ever-continuing environmental changes are not readily altered," Dr. Benson points out, "better prevention and perhaps therapy of related diseases such as hypertension might be achieved by altering the autonomic responses of an individual to his environment . . .

It is hoped that conditioning techniques [biofeedback] will be of value in altering autonomic nervous system responses which might result in and also which might perpetuate hypertension."

Conceivably, as the technique is refined and becomes better understood and more readily teachable, it may eliminate the need for drug treatment in at least some patients, reduce drug needs in others, and perhaps even be useful as a means of preventing hypertension.

SORTING OUT HYPERTENSIVES:
HIGH AND LOW RISKS

A small group of hypertensive patients defy all the statistics by continuing in good health despite blood pressure levels that would prove detrimental to others.

A possible explanation which, if true, could have great practical value, has been proposed by Dr. John Laragh and his colleagues at the Presbyterian Hospital in New York City. Their theory is that such people have low levels of renin in their blood.

Renin we have seen is a compound produced by the kidneys in response to a fall in blood pressure. Once it moves from the kidneys into the blood, renin starts up a series of chemical events that tend to increase the body's retention of water. The greater volume of water increases the volume of blood and, with the increased blood volume, blood pressure rises.

Renin production by the kidneys is part of the body's control mechanism. It helps to assure that a proper level of blood pressure is maintained so that blood circulates adequately.

Normally, the kidneys stop producing renin when the low blood pressure condition is corrected. But if the shutoff signal is not obeyed and the kidneys continue to produce renin, chronic hypertension may ensue.

The findings of Dr. Laragh and his colleagues suggest

that, in fact, there may be two forms of hypertension. In one, the amounts of renin in the blood are low and this form of hypertension may be truly benign. In patients they have been studying, the investigators have not been able to find one with low blood renin—about a quarter of some 200 patients who have been thoroughly investigated—who has suffered a heart attack or stroke.

In contrast, 14 percent of those with high renin levels, plus even 11 percent of those with normal renin levels, suffered either a heart attack or a stroke.

It seems significant, too, that on the average, patients in the low renin group were older and had had hypertension longer than the others. Since they were older and had had the elevated pressures longer, it would have been expected that they would have been more likely to have suffered heart attacks or strokes.

Therefore, provided the findings can be confirmed by further research on a much larger scale, high blood pressure patients with low blood renin may need less drug treatment whereas those with high renin activity may benefit from earlier and more aggressive treatment.

Another possibility is that the finding could lead to the development of antihypertensive drugs that specifically reduce blood levels of renin, and such drugs are already being sought.

HYPERTENSION IS A PROBLEM
WHOSE TIME HAS COME

The developments in this chapter reflect only a small portion of the new pathways now being explored.

In the future, hypertension control will be even further simplified; new and even better-targeted drugs will become available; and drugless treatments may become broadly effective.

Hypertension is a problem whose time has come—not only in the sense that its importance as a killer and crippler has been recognized, which in turn has led to increased research efforts that will pay off in the future; it is immediately controllable, with effective measures available now.

It would be tragic to wait—and waste—a generation for future refinements.

Hypertension will be on the run only when we use our existing knowledge and measures.

If you have hypertension, your future is right now.

CAMPAIGNS

Vast campaigns to find people with high blood pressure and get them into treatment have been recommended by authorities, and many are under way.

Late in 1971, The Inter-Society Commission for Heart Disease Resources, representing 29 leading medical and nursing organizations, urged that everyone between the ages of 15 and 65 be screened for hypertension. It recommended that detection programs be sponsored by labor and management groups, that screening programs be set up in community centers, in mobile units, or through door-to-door surveys.

It recommended that each community organize its own system of care for hypertensive patients. One level would be composed of various facilities for ambulatory care, including doctors' offices, hospital outpatient clinics, industrial medical programs, and neighborhood health centers. These units would be supplemented by a Neighborhood Hypertension Unit designed to perform much of the routine follow-up physicians might not have time to do. A trained health worker would even be sent into the homes of patients who do not keep appointments.

At the NASA Goddard Space Flight Center, where over the last five years the death rate from heart and blood vessel diseases has increased from 5 to 14 per 10,000 employees, an intensive program is under way. Any employee in whom hypertension is suspected must return on three successive days for repeat blood pressure checks. If the hypertension is confirmed, he is referred to a physician of his choice for treatment and is requested to return to the NASA medical facility at regular intervals, in some cases even daily, until the adequacy of treatment has been established.

Turning up hypertensives is not enough. The medical students and high-schoolers who were trained at Tulane University School of Medicine for three weeks (see Chapter 4) did more than ring doorbells and take measurements. They gave every hypertensive they found a yellow card to report for treatment at a local hospital that had agreed to do the treating. The hospital has almost two million outpatient visits a year; it figured another 3,000 wouldn't be all that difficult to take.

The Tulane survey cost $5,000. Some authorities are arguing that the 100 medical schools in the United States be given grants of $5,000 each for similar programs, which might turn up as many as 400,000 currently untreated cases of hypertension. "I don't know how else you could save so many lives for so little money," says Dr. F. Gilbert McMahon of Tulane who conceived and directed the project.

"Our hypertension survey in New Orleans was an eye-opener in many ways," Dr. McMahon adds. "Among other things, it made me wonder if our priorities aren't badly mixed up. Not long ago I read that someone has advocated spending several million dollars in an all-out war on tuberculosis, which kills about 5,000 persons each year. That same number die of heart disease and stroke every two days!

"Again, vast sums are spent each year on diabetes-detection programs yielding one or two previously undiagnosed cases per hundred screened. Even after diabetes is detected, there still remains the question as to the extent that treatment which is presently available can retard cardiovascular-renal (heart, blood vessel and kidney) and eye complications.

"In contrast, hypertension screening can identify 36 cases per 100, as we demonstrated. . . . It can be done at extremely low cost. And there are many drugs that reduce blood pressure and thus prolong the useful lives of most subjects."

In a report in a professional journal, *Medical Opinion,*

Dr. McMahon goes on to say: "Perhaps one reason that the detection of hypertension has attracted so little attention is that other aspects of cardiovascular disease are more spectacular. Each year, millions of dollars are spent in such areas as cardiac transplant, mechanical hearts, coronary-care units, etc. This work is important and merits support. But I believe that when we think only in terms of exchanging new hearts for old, or of keeping old hearts beating in coronary-care units, we do not even scratch the surface. Although we thereby may save a few lives, close to 1,200,000 people will continue to die each year from heart disease and stroke.

"The only way to bring about a sizeable reduction in this terrible toll is early identification and adequate, persistent treatment of persons at high risk.

"It is now documented that lowering blood pressure can bring about substantial reductions in mortality and morbidity of hypertensive patients. Particularly impressive is the fact that even mild hypertension carries added risk. One well-known study has shown that the mortality of patients with elevated blood pressures is directly related to the degree of elevation. In a large group of subjects first studied at age 45, almost 22 percent of those with pressures of 160/100 were dead at the end of ten years. Of those with pressures of 152/95, about 17 percent had died. When the pressure was 152/85, the death rate fell to 13.7 percent. . . .

"The fact that antihypertensive medication will reduce morbidity and mortality was amply demonstrated in a VA study. . . . With conclusive evidence that the disease is treatable and that treatment saves lives, it would seem that we should be waging all-out war on hypertension."

In Bergen County, New Jersey, health workers have started a pilot program which, if successful, could make dentists an important factor in reducing the toll of deaths from hypertension. Actually, a few Bergen County dentists had taken the unusual step of measuring the blood pressure of all of their patients. Now, through the cooperation of the Bergen County medical and dental societies, other dentists and dental technicians as well are learning how to take blood pressures in a special training program. The aim is to detect undiagnosed cases.

In New York City, where as many as two million people may have hypertension, the Department of Health in May 1972, although pressed for funds, decided to tackle the problem anyhow. The Department operates 25 tuberculosis clinics and 14 venereal disease clinics, along with maternal and infant care clinics. All told, through these clinics yearly pass some 150,000 people. Now, whatever their reason for visiting a clinic, they are being screened for high blood pressure. Anyone with elevated pressure is checked again the same day. If the pressure is still elevated, there is a third check 48 to 72 hours later. If the third check is still positive, the patient is referred for treatment, to his own physician or to a Health Department clinic in a hospital, or to the outpatient department of any of a number of voluntary hospitals cooperating with the program. The Health Department follows up, checking with hospital clinics to make certain referred patients turn up for treatment, and contacting any who do not turn up.

The New York City program has more than the obvious purpose of finding and treating previously undiagnosed and untreated hypertensives among the people coming to its TB, VD, and other clinics. "We are trying," says Dr. Joseph Cimino, New York City Health Commissioner, "to convert both the public and the medical community to believing in long-term treatment of hypertension. We can't treat all the hypertensives in New York City. What we have to do is convince the medical community that those individuals doctors see with hypertension should be treated. We are trying to increase pressure on all physicians for hypertensives to be treated seriously and adequately."

The National Heart and Lung Institute has set up, as of "highest immediate priority," a Hypertension Detection and Follow-up Program. Fifteen clinical centers across the country—in Washington, D.C., Salt Lake City, Birmingham, Chicago, Boston, Baltimore, Los Angeles, and elsewhere— are each screening 8,000 to 12,000 persons aged 30 to 69, to detect the estimated 800 to 1,000 or more who would be expected to have hypertension. Those with hypertension will, of course, be offered treatment.

But the program has other vital purposes. It is seeking to determine the most effective ways of getting people interested in being tested for hypertension. And, beyond that, it is seeking means to motivate people with hypertension to take it seriously, despite lack of symptoms, and continue with treatment rather than drop out.

To get people to allow themselves to be screened for hypertension, the centers are testing various approaches: cold-turkey door-to-door visits, door-to-door visits preceded by letter, going into factories, setting up mobile screening vans in churches, shopping centers, and other neighborhood gathering places.

Efforts to find ways to reduce the dropout-from-treatment rate, which began even before the program was set up, are continuing.

For example, one of the hypertension clinics in the National Heart and Lung Institute program is housed at the District of Columbia General Hospital in Washington, D.C. There, for 20 years, Dr. Frank A. Finnerty, Jr., referred to earlier in the study on blacks, has had a 42 percent dropout rate. Not long ago Dr. Finnerty and his co-workers decided to do a study to find the reasons for the dropout rate in hypertension clinics. Clinics at the District of Columbia General Hospital, Washington Hospital Center, Columbia Hospital, and Georgetown University Medical Center were covered. All dropouts in a 5-week period at all the clinics were interviewed in depth.

It turned out that there was some confusion about the seriousness of hypertension. Ninety-five percent of the dropouts recognized that hypertension was more serious than a cold; 44 percent considered it as important as diabetes; 71 percent considered it as important as heart disease; whereas 13 percent felt it was about as important as influenza.

Waiting time was a major criticism of 63 percent of the dropouts. At some clinics, the average waiting time prior to examination by the doctor was 2½ hours and, after examination, an average waiting time of 1.8 hours at the pharmacy.

For all the long waiting, the average time a patient spent
with a physician was only 7½ minutes. At some clinics, the
poor doctor-patient relationship was made worse by the fact
that a different physician saw the patient on each visit. Economic costs were not a major problem; in fact, 78.5 percent
of patients received economic support for medical care.

Finnerty and his study group concluded that patients
dropped out of the clinics not for a lack of intelligence, dis-
regard for their health, or economic reasons; on the con-
trary, the dropouts were an intelligent, concerned group
whose motivation was limited by time and a system they
saw as not very concerned with them. The study group also
concluded that there was need not only for a major reduction in time patients have to spend in clinics but also for a
relationship that recognizes the desire of patients to know
more about their disease and its treatment and a staff that
recognizes the patients' perceptiveness and concern with
their own well-being.

At Finnerty's own clinic, in an attempt to reduce the dropout rate, a reorganization was put into effect. As a patient
is put into long-term treatment, he is assigned to a doctor
and a health aide who are his source of contact and care.
Patients are examined at all times by the same aide and
physician. Night and weekend coverage by telephone is
available. The appointment system provides for the clinic
visit on a convenient schedule, and each patient is called
prior to his visit to remind him of the appointment. Medication is provided by the clinic. Since the reorganization,
the dropout rate has been reduced from 42 percent to 8 percent.

In July 1972, the Veterans Administration began what
will become a massive hypertension detection and treatment
program. It aims to screen and provide suitable treatment
where needed for every one of the 28 million living veterans
in the country, and then to reach out to families of veterans
and to stimulate community programs.

The VA system is the largest health care system in operation in the country. It has 168 hospitals with almost 100,000

beds, 202 independent clinics, 63 nursing homes, a staff of some 150,000 physicians, dentists, nurses, and every category of health professional. Its network of facilities and people is located not more than 100 miles, or a two-hour drive, from 90 percent of all veterans. On any given day, the VA system is treating 160,000 people.

The VA hypertension program started in a dozen of the large VA hospitals with long experience in hypertension research. There, techniques for screening and treatment follow-up are being put to the test and any bugs are being eliminated. The program then will be extended to all the 168 hospitals in the system. Initially, all veterans receiving any kind of medical care at VA institutions will be checked for hypertension. Then all other veterans in the service area of each hospital will be urged to have blood pressures checked.

Although the VA has no legislative authority to treat anyone other than veterans, it sees an urgent need to expand its hypertension program beyond veterans alone. To do this it has sought and obtained assurances of cooperation from various service organizations, heart association chapters, and county medical societies.

With the cooperation of such organizations and societies, the VA plans to extend hypertension screening examinations to veterans' families and to large portions of the general population in communities where its facilities are located, with VA physicians, nurses, and other personnel volunteering their services during off-duty hours.

In a demonstration of the importance of seeking out hypertension, the VA took the blood pressures of 500 men attending special meetings of the American Legion and the Veterans of Foreign Wars in Washington recently. Thirty-nine percent of the men were found to have hypertension, and half of them, all men with some knowledge of medical affairs and often concerned with the medical service provided for veterans, had no previous knowledge that they were hypertensive.

Treatment

Appendix

ANTIHYPERTENSIVE DRUGS

Trade name	Generic drug name
Diuretics	
Anhydron	cyclothiazide
Benuron	bendroflumethiazide
Diuril	chlorothiazide
Enduron	methyclorthiazide
Esidrix	hydrochlorothiazide
Exna	benzthiazide
Hydro DIURIL	hydrochlorothiazide
Hydromox	quinethazone
Hygroton	chlorthalidone
Naturetin	bendroflumethiazide
Oretic	hydrochlorothiazide
Renese	polythiazide
Saluron	hydroflumethiazide
Ganglion blockers	
Ansolysen	pentolinium
Inversine	mecamylamine
Veratrum	
Veralba	protoveratrine
Rauwolfia and Reserpine	
Eskaserp Spansule	reserpine, time-released
Harmonyl	deserpidine
Moderil	rescinnamine
Raudixin	whole root

Rauwiloid   alseroxylon
Sandril, Serpasil   reserpine
Singoserp   syrosingopine

Others
Aldomet   methyldopa
Apresoline   hydralazine
Ismelin   guanethidine

Combinations
Butiserpazide   reserpine, hydrochlorothiazide,
                        butabarbital
Butiserpine   reserpine, butabarbital
Diupres   reserpine, chlorothiazide
Enduronyl   deserpidine, methyclothiazide
Exna-R   reserpine, benzythiazide
Hydromox-R   reserpine, quinethazone
Hydropres   reserpine, hydrochlorothiazide
Metatensin   reserpine, trichlormethiazide
Naquival   reserpine, trichlormethiazide
Rautrax-N   rauwolfia, bendroflumethiazide,
                        potassium chloride
Rauzide   rauwolfia, bendroflumethiazide
Regroton   reserpine, chlorthalidone
Renese-R   reserpine, polythiazide
Salutensin   reserpine, hydroflumethiazide,
                        protoveratrine A (veratrum)
Ser-Ap-Es   reserpine, hydralazine,
                        hydrochlorothiazide
Serpasil Apresoline reserpine, hydralazine
Serpasil-Esidrix   reserpine, hydrochlorothiazide
Solfo-Serpine   reserpine, phenobarbital

Courtesy American Heart Association ("Drug Treatment of Arterial Hypertension") and *Medical Annals of the District of Columbia,* January, 1969
("Drug Therapy of Hypertension").

2nd part

FOODS HIGH IN SALT (SODIUM)

Meat, Meat Flavorings, and Fish
Anchovies
Bacon
Bacon fat
Caviar
Chipped beef
Corned beef
Dried cod
Frankfurters
Ham
Herring
Luncheon meats
Meat extracts
Meat sauces
Meat tenderizers
Salt pork
Salted and smoked fish
Salted and smoked meats
Sardines
Sausages

Appetizers, Sauces, and Seasonings
Cheeses
Celery salt
Chili sauce
Garlic salt
Ketchup
Mustard
Olives
Onion salt
Pickles
Potato chips
Pretzels
Regular bouillon cubes
Relishes

Salted nuts
Salted popcorn
Sauerkraut
Soy sauce
Table salt
Worcestershire sauce

Courtesy Standard Brands, Inc. (*Low Sodium Diets Can Be Delicious*).

FOODS MODERATELY HIGH
IN SALT (SODIUM)

Breads
Breads *
Rolls *
Crackers *
Waffles *

Vegetables
Beets
Beet greens
Canned vegetables *
Canned vegetable juices *
Carrots
Celery
Swiss chard
Dandelion and mustard greens
Kale
Spinach

Meat and fish
Canned meats *
Clams
Crabs
Kidneys
Lobsters
Oysters
Scallops

* Usually commercial.

Shrimp

Fats and oils
Salad dressings *
Salted butter
Salted margarine

Other
Beverage mixes *
Baking powder
Molasses

* Usually commercial.
Courtesy Standard Brands, Inc. (*Low Sodium Diets Can Be Delicious*).

DAILY DIET PLAN * IN UNITS FOR MILD,ᵃ MODERATE,ᵇ AND STRICTᶜ SODIUM RESTRICTION WITH VARYING CALORIC NEEDS

An exchange system based on seven food lists developed by the American Heart Association is utilized here. In addition to varying levels of sodium restriction, provision is made for supplying different caloric needs while meeting other nutrient requirements. Each dietary regimen calls for a definite number of units from each food list, as detailed in the table preceding the food lists. With the prescribed daily diet plan and the accompanying food lists, the patient may then select his foods for the day and arrange them into menus. The sodium content of drinking and cooking water must be included in computing the daily sodium intake. Information on water analyses can usually be obtained from the local Department of Health.

GENERAL RULES: (1) Avoid the use of salt at the table and of soda, monosodium glutamate (MSG), and baking powder in food preparation. (2) Avoid laxatives or other medications containing sodium salts. (3) Do not use water from a home water softener for drinking or cooking, as these appliances add sodium to the water.

The number of units you are allowed for each list depends upon which diet plan your doctor has prescribed for you.

The *1,200-calorie diet plan* is a reducing diet. The *1,800-calorie diet plan* is like the 1,200-calorie diet, but with more bread, fat, and free choice units. The *unrestricted calorie diet plan* allows the greatest freedom of the three.

So—no matter which of the three diet plans your doctor has prescribed—you will have all the nutrients you need as well as the number of calories and the amount of sodium you may have *if you follow your diet plan exactly*. If you add foods that are not on the lists, or increase quantities, you will be adding sodium or calories; if you omit foods, or eat less than the specified amount, you will be leaving out important parts of your diet.

Every day you are to have a definite number of *units* from each list.

---

* From the *Merck Manual*, twelfth edition, © 1972 Merck & Co., Inc., Rahway, New Jersey.

  ᵃ *Mild*—Salt foods lightly during preparation; use no salt at table.
  ᵇ *Moderate*—Only ¼ tsp of salt/day may be used (in food preparation or at the table).
  ᶜ *Strict*—Prepare and eat all foods without salt.

Examples of units, taken from the fruit list, are 1 apple, 1 cup strawberries, ½ cup applesauce, and 10 cherries.

Food List No.	Unrestricted Calories	1,800 Calories	1,200 Calories
1	2 units	2 units	0 units
1A	0	0	2
2A	1 or more	1 or more	1 or more
2B	1 or more	1	1
2C	1 or more	1	1
3	2 or more	4	4
4	4 or more	7	5
5	5	5	5
6	as desired	4	0
7	as desired	2	1

FOOD LISTS FOR SODIUM-RESTRICTED DIETS

LIST 1—MILK PRODUCTS

	List 1	List 1A
FOR MILD SODIUM RESTRICTION	1,800 or Unrestricted Calorie Diet Each unit contains approx.: Carbohydrate 12, protein 8, fat 10 gm; calories 170; sodium 120 mg 1 unit = 1 cup Whole milk 1 cup Whole milk buttermilk 1 cup Evaporated whole milk (reconstituted) 2 Fat units plus 1 cup Nonfat buttermilk 2 Fat units plus 3 tbsp Nonfat dry milk (or amt. (powder) specified on package for making 1 cup) 2 Fat units plus 1 cup Nonfat dry milk (reconstituted) 2 Fat units plus 1 cup Skim milk *N.B.:* 2 units from the Meat list may be substituted for not more than 1 Milk unit/day. AVOID: Any commercial foods made of milk—ice cream, sherbet, milk shakes, chocolate milk, malted milk, milk mixes, condensed milk etc.	1,200-Calorie Diet Each unit contains approx.: Carbohydrate 12, protein 8 gm; fat negligible; calories 85; sodium 120 mg 1 unit = 1 cup Skim milk 1 cup Evaporated skim milk (reconstituted) 1 cup Nonfat buttermilk 3 tbsp Nonfat dry milk (or amt. (powder) specified on package for making 1 cup) 1 cup Nonfat dry milk (reconstituted) *N.B.:* 1 unit from the Meat list may be substituted for not more than 1 Milk unit/day. AVOID: Whole milk or any commercial foods made of milk—ice cream, sherbet, milk shakes, chocolate milk, malted milk, milk mixes, condensed milk, etc.
FOR MODERATE & STRICT SODIUM RESTRICTION	As above except that buttermilk must be unsalted. Where less than 500 mg of sodium is necessary, use special low sodium milk products.	As above except that buttermilk must be unsalted. Where less than 500 mg of sodium is necessary, use special low-sodium dry milk products; avoid buttermilk products.

LIST 2–VEGETABLES

	Group A	Group B	Group C
FOR MILD SODIUM RESTRICTION	Each unit contains: Carbohydrate, protein, fat, and calories negligible; sodium varies	Each unit contains approx.: Carbohydrate 7, protein 2, fat 0 gm; calories 35; sodium 9 mg	Each unit contains approx.: Carbohydrate 15, protein 2, fat 0 gm; calories 70; sodium 5 mg

Group A	Group B	Group C	
1 unit = ½ cup	1 unit = ½ cup	1 unit =	
Artichoke	Beets	¼ cup	Beans, baked (no pork)
Asparagus	Carrots		
Beet greens	Onions	½ cup cooked	Beans, lima or navy (fresh or dried)
Broccoli	Peas		
Brussels sprouts	Pumpkin		
Cabbage	Rutabaga (yellow turnip)	⅓ cup or ½ small ear	Corn
Cauliflower			
Celery	Squash, winter (acorn, Hubbard, etc.)	½ cup	Hominy
Chard, Swiss		½ cup cooked	Lentils (dried)
Chicory	Turnip, white		
Cucumber			
Dandelion greens		⅔ cup	Parsnips
Eggplant		½ cup cooked	Peas, split green or yellow, cowpeas, etc. (dried)
Endive			
Escarole			
Green beans			
Kale		1 small	Potato, white
Lettuce		½ cup	Potatoes, mashed
Mushrooms			
Mustard greens			
Okra		¼ cup or ½ small	Sweet potato
Peppers, green or red			
Radishes			
Spinach			
Squash, summer (yellow, zucchini, etc.)			
Tomato juice	*N.B.:* 2 units from Group A may be substituted for 1 unit from Group B.	*N.B.:* 1 unit from the Bread list may be substituted for 1 unit from Group C.	
Tomatoes			
Turnip greens			
Wax beans			

	Group A	Group B	Group C
FOR MODERATE & STRICT SODIUM RESTRICTION	All of the above, except artichokes, beet greens, celery, chard, dandelion greens, kale, mustard greens, spinach.	All of the above, except beets, carrots, turnips.	All of the above, except hominy.

Canned vegetables and tomato juice should be of low-sodium dietetic type. Frozen vegetables must be processed without salt. (Check labels.)

LIST 3—FRUIT PRODUCTS

FOR ALL SODIUM-RESTRICTED DIETS	Includes fresh, frozen, canned, or dried fruit Each unit contains approx.: Carbohydrate 10 gm; protein and fat negligible; calories 40; sodium 2 mg

1 unit =

1 cup	Blackberries, raspberries, strawberries, watermelon
⅔ cup	Blueberries
⅓ cup	Apple juice or cider, cranberry juice (sweetened), pineapple juice
½ cup	Applesauce, fruit cup or mixed fruits, diced pineapple; orange, tangerine, or grapefruit juice
¼ cup	Apricot nectar, grape juice, prune juice
1	Apple, fig, pear, tangerine, orange, peach
2	Apricots (fresh or dried), dates, plums, prunes
½	Banana, grapefruit, mango
10	Cherries
12	Grapes
⅓	Papaya
¼	Cantaloupe
⅛	Honeydew melon
1 tbsp	Cranberries (sweetened)
2 tbsp	Raisins, rhubarb (sweetened)

Fresh lemons and limes, unsweetened cranberries, cranberry juice, and rhubarb: Use as desired; do not count as a unit.

On 1,200- and 1,800-calorie diets, do not use glazed or sweetened fruits or those packed in sugar syrup.

LIST 4—BREAD AND CEREAL PRODUCTS

FOR MILD SODIUM RESTRICTION	Each unit contains approx.: Carbohydrate 15, protein 2 gm; fat negligible; calories 70; sodium 5 mg *N.B.:* 1 unit from the Vegetable list, Group C, may be substituted for 1 Bread unit.

1 unit =

1 slice	Bread
4 pieces (3½″ × 1½″ × ⅛″)	Melba toast
1 medium	Roll, biscuit, or muffin
1 cube (1½″)	Cornbread
2 3″	Griddle cakes
½ cup (cooked)	Farina, grits, oatmeal, rolled wheat, wheat meal (lightly salted)
⅔ biscuit	Shredded wheat
¾ cup	Other dry cereal
1½ tbsp	Uncooked barley
2 tbsp	Cornmeal
5 2″ square	Crackers (low-sodium dietetic)
2½ tbsp	Flour or cornstarch
2	Graham crackers
½ cup cooked	Macaroni, rice (brown or white), noodles, or spaghetti
1 5″ square	Matzo (plain, unsalted)
1½ cups	Popcorn
2 tbsp uncooked	Tapioca
1 3″ square section	Waffle, yeast

FOR MODERATE & STRICT SODIUM RESTRICTION	As above except that yeast bread and rolls, quick breads, and cooked cereals must be made without salt or monosodium glutamate; all breads must be made with sodium-free baking powder or low-sodium dietetic mix, and the dry cereal used must have not more than 6 mg of sodium/100 gm of cereal (check the label). Avoid self-rising cornmeal; graham crackers; salted popcorn, potato chips, pretzels, and crackers.

Appendix

LIST 5—MEAT OR MEAT SUBSTITUTES

FOR
MILD
SODIUM
RESTRICTION

Each unit contains approx.:
Carbohydrate negligible; protein 7, fat 5 gm; calories 75; sodium 25 mg

1 unit =

1 oz, cooked

Beef	Lamb	Rabbit
Brain	Liver (beef, calf,	Tongue
Chicken	chicken, pork)	Turkey
Duck	Pork	Veal
Kidney	Quail	

Bass	Eels	Salmon
Blueqsh	Flounder	Scallops
Catfish	Halibut	Shrimp
Clams	Lobster	Sole
Cod	Oyster	Trout
Crab	Rockfish	Tuna

1oz	American cheddar or Swiss cheese
¼ cup	Cottage cheese (lightly salted)
1	Egg
2 tbsp	Low-sodium dietetic peanut butter

AVOID: Salty or smoked meats or fish (e.g., bacon, luncheon meats, chipped or corned beef, ham, frankfurters, salt pork, smoked tongue, sausage; anchovies, caviar, salted and dried cod, herring, sardines, etc.), processed cheese, cheese spreads, Roquefort, Camembert, Gorgonzola.

FOR
MODERATE &
STRICT
RESTRICTION

As above except that (1) brain, kidney, and shellfish are to be avoided. (2) Canned meat, poultry, and fish are to be of low-sodium dietetic type. (3) Cottage cheese should be unsalted; other cheeses are to be of low-sodium dietetic type. (4) Fish, except as noted under (2), to be fresh only. (5) Eggs are limited to 1/day.

LIST 6—FATS

FOR
MILD
SODIUM
RESTRICTION

Each unit contains approx.:
Fat 5 gm; calories 45; sodium negligible

1 unit =

⅛ 4" diameter	Avocado
1 tsp (1 pat)	Butter or margarine
1 tbsp	Cream, heavy (sweet or sour)
2 tbsp	Cream, light (sweet or sour)
1 tsp	Fat or oil, cooking
1 tbsp	French dressing
1 tsp	Mayonnaise
6 small	Nuts, unsalted

AVOID: Salted nuts, bacon and bacon fat, olives, salt pork.

FOR
MODERATE &
STRICT
SODIUM
RESTRICTION

As above except that salted butter and margarine are to be avoided; commercial salads and dressings are to be low-sodium dietetic type.

LIST 7—FREE CHOICE

FOR **MILD** **SODIUM** **RESTRICTION**	1 unit from	List 4—Breads
	75 calories	Candy (made without salted nuts)
	2 units from	List 6—Fats
	2 units from	List 3—Fruits
	4 tsp	Sugar (white or brown)
	4 tsp	Syrup, honey, jelly, jam, or marmalade
	1 unit from	List 2—Vegetables, Group C

Flavorings and seasonings may be used as desired except that barbecue sauce, bouillon, catsup, celery salt, chili sauce, garlic salt, prepared horseradish, meat extracts or tenderizers, monosodium glutamate, prepared mustard, olives, onion salt, pickles, radishes, soy sauce, Worcestershire sauce, and cooking wines are to be avoided.

FOR
MODERATE &
STRICT
SODIUM
RESTRICTION

As above except that candy is to be homemade, salt-free, or low-sodium dietetic.

MENUS FOR MILD SODIUM RESTRICTION
(COURTESY AMERICAN HEART ASSOCIATION)
If you are on the 1,200-calorie diet

Breakfast

½ cup orange juice
½ cup oatmeal   ½ cup skim milk
2 teaspoons sugar*
1 slice toast   Coffee or tea, if desired

Midmorning snack:
  1 slice toast
  2 teaspoons jelly *
  Coffee or tea, if desired

Lunch

Tomato and fish salad *made with:*
2 ounces tuna or salmon
1 medium tomato
1-2 leaves of lettuce
5 crackers (two-inch squares)
1 medium peach
½ cup skim milk   Coffee or tea, if desired

Midafternoon snack:
  ½ cup skim milk

Dinner

3-ounce beef patty
½ cup whipped potato   ½ cup green peas
Cole slaw with low-calorie dressing
1 medium roll
½ cup fruit cup   Coffee or tea, if desired

Evening snack:
  ½ cup skim milk
  1 small apple   * Selected as free choice

Breakfast

Half grapefruit

1 poached egg   2 slices toast

1 small pat butter °

½ cup skim milk   Coffee or tea, if desired

Midmorning snack:
½ cup skim milk

Lunch

Cream of vegetable soup with chicken *made with:*
½ cup of mixed vegetables from Groups A and B
⅓ cup corn (from Group C)
½ cup skim milk
1 ounce (2 tablespoons) diced chicken
Lettuce salad with low-calorie dressing
1 slice toast

2 small slices pineapple   Coffee or tea, if desired

Midafternoon snack:
2 medium plums

Dinner

3 ounces broiled steak
Mushrooms, as desired

6 asparagus spears   ½ cup summer squash

1 medium corn muffin   1 small pat butter °

2 apricots   Coffee or tea, if desired

Evening snack:
½ cup skim milk:
1 slice bread   ° Selected as free choice

For the 1,800-calorie diet

Breakfast

2 medium prunes with 2 tablespoons juice
¾ cup puffed wheat   1 cup milk
1 slice toast   1 small pat butter
Coffee or tea, if desired

Midmorning snack:
½ cup milk

Lunch

2 ounces broiled liver
Baked acorn squash with 1 small pat butter
Cabbage slaw with caraway seeds, green pepper, and vinegar
2 medium muffins   1 small pat butter
Apricot bread pudding *made with:*
1 slice bread   *4 dried apricot halves*
¼ cup milk   *1 small pat butter*
Coffee or tea, if desired

Midafternoon snack:
1 small orange

Dinner

Baked casserole of beef with whipped potato topping *made with:*
3 ounces cooked beef
½ cup broth from beef
½ cup potato
Green beans
Tomato and cucumber salad on lettuce leaf
with 1 tablespoon French dressing *
2 medium rolls   1 small pat butter *
½ grapefruit
Coffee or tea, if desired

Evening snack:
1 small sliced banana * with
¼ cup milk   * Selected as free choice

Breakfast

½ cup grapefruit juice
1 medium egg, scrambled
½ cup applesauce
2 slices toast   1 small pat butter
Coffee or tea, if desired

Midmorning snack:
  ½ cup milk
  5 crackers (two-inch squares)

Lunch

2 ounces sliced roast chicken
⅓ cup bread dressing
1 tablespoon cranberry sauce
½ cup cauliflower   Lettuce salad
1 medium roll   I small pat butter
1 cup milk   Coffee or tea, if desired

Midafternoon snack:
  1 small pear
  Coffee or tea, if desired

Dinner

Homemade bean soup
made with ½ cup cooked dried beans
2 ounces broiled halibut with lemon
½ cup green peas   1 small broiled tomato
½ baked sweet potato *
1 small cornmeal muffin   2 small pats butter
Rice-raisin pudding *made with:*
½ *cup cooked rice*
2 *tablespoons raisins**
½ *cup milk*
Coffee or tea, if desired

Evening snack:
  12 grapes *
  Coffee or tea, if deisred   * Selected as free choice

If you are on the unrestricted calorie diet

. . . take a vacation from meal planning with these sample menus.

Breakfast

Grapefruit sections
Farina
Sweet rolls or pancakes
Butter   Sugar   Syrup
Milk   Coffee or tea, if desired
Midmorning snack, if desired:
  Banana

Lunch

Tomato juice
Roast loin of pork   Applesauce
Boiled potato   Turnip greens
Radishes
Corn muffins   Butter
Coffee or tea, if desired
Midafternoon snack, if desired:
  Grapes

Dinner

Meat loaf
Creole sauce
Stewed corn   Broccoli with lemon butter
Fresh fruit salad with mayonnaise
Biscuits   Butter
Caramel custard
Coffee or tea, if desired
Evening snack:
  1 cup milk
  Cookies, if desired

Breakfast

Cantaloupe
Shredded Wheat
Boiled egg

Toast   Butter
Jelly   Sugar
Milk   Coffee or tea, if desired

Midmorning snack, if desired:
  Sweet rolls
  Coffee or tea

Lunch

Broiled lamb patty
Mint jelly

Rice   Stewed tomatoes and okra
Roll   Butter
Orange whip with orange sections
Coffee or tea, if desired

Midafternoon snack, if desired:
  Lemonade with sugar
  Cookies

Dinner

Homemade barley soup
Sliced roast beef   Mushroom sauce
Baked potato   Green peas
Sweet-sour cabbage
Rolls
Cherry pie   Coffee or tea, if desired

Evening snack:
  Milk
  Cookies, if desired

**A FAT-CONTROLLED, LOW CHOLESTEROL MEAL PLAN TO
REDUCE THE RISK OF HEART ATTACK**

Every day, select foods from each of the basic food groups in lists
1–6, and follow the recommendations for number and size of servings.

1 MEAT • POULTRY • FISH DRIED BEANS and PEAS NUTS • EGGS

1 serving . . . 3–4 ounces of cooked meat or fish (not
including bone or fat) or 3–4 ounces of a vegetable
listed here

Use 2 or more servings (a total of 6–8 ounces) daily

RECOMMENDED

AVOID OR USE SPARINGLY

**Chicken • turkey • veal • fish •
most of your meat meals for
the week.**
Shellfish: clams • crabs • lobster
• oysters • scallops • shrimp •
are low in fat but high in
cholesterol. Use a 4-ounce
serving as a substitute for meat
no more than twice a week.

Duck • goose

**Beef • lamb • pork • ham • in
no more than 5 meals per week.**
Choose lean ground meat and
lean cuts of meat • trim all
visible fat before cooking • bake,
broil, roast, or stew so that you
can discard the fat which cooks
out of the meat.

Heavily marbled and fatty meats •
spare ribs • mutton • frankfurters • sausage • fatty ham-
burgers • bacon • luncheon meats.

Nuts and dried beans and peas:
Kidney beans • lima beans baked
beans • lentils • chick peas
(garbanzos) • split peas • are
high in vegetable protein and
may be used in place of meat
occasionally.
Egg whites as desired.

Organ meats: liver • kidney •
heart • sweetbreads • are very
high in cholesterol. Since liver is
very rich in vitamins and iron, it
should not be eliminated from the
diet completely. Use a 4-ounce
serving in a meat meal no more
than once a week.

Egg yolks: limit to 3 per week
including eggs used in cooking.
Cakes, batters, sauces, and other
foods containing egg yolks.

2 VEGETABLES and FRUIT

(Fresh, frozen, or canned)

1 serving . . . ½ cup
Use at least 4 servings daily

RECOMMENDED

One serving should be a source of vitamin C:
Broccoli • cabbage (raw) • tomatoes. Berries • cantaloupe • grapefruit (or juice) • mango • melon • orange (or juice) • papaya • strawberries • tangerines.

One serving should be a source of vitamin A—dark green leafy or yellow vegetables, or yellow fruits:
Broccoli • carrots • chard • chicory • escarole • greens (beet, collard, dandelion, mustard, turnip) • kale • peas • rutabagas • spinach • string beans • sweet potatoes and yams • watercress • winter squash • yellow corn. Apricots • cantaloupe • mango • papaya.

Other vegetables and fruits are also very nutritious; they should be eaten in salads, main dishes, snacks, and desserts, *in addition* to the recommended daily allowances of high vitamin A and C vegetables and fruits.

AVOID OR USE SPARINGLY

Olives and avocados are very high in fat calories and should be used in moderation.

If you must limit your calories, use vegetables such as potatoes, corn, or lima beans sparingly. To add variety to your diet, one serving (½ cup) of any one of these may be substituted for one serving of bread of cereals.

3 BREAD and CEREALS

(Whole grain, enriched, or restored)

1 serving of bread . . . 1 slice
1 serving of cereal . . .
½ cup, cooked
1 cup, cold with skimmed milk

Use at least 4 servings daily

RECOMMENDED	AVOID OR USE SPARINGLY
Breads made with a minimum of saturated fat:	Butter rolls • commercial biscuits, muffins, doughnuts, sweet rolls, cakes, crackers • egg bread, cheese bread • commercial mixes containing dried eggs and whole milk.
White enriched (including raisin bread) • whole wheat • English muffins • French bread • Italian bread• oatmeal bread • pumpernickel rye bread.	
Biscuits, muffins, and griddle cakes made at home, using an allowed liquid oil as shortening.	
Cereal (hot and cold) • rice • melba toast • matzo • pretzels.	
Pasta: macaroni • noodles (except egg noodles) • spaghetti.	

4 MILK PRODUCTS

1 serving ... 8 ounces (1 cup)

Buy only skimmed milk that has been fortified with vitamins A and D.

Daily servings:
Children up to 12 ... 3 or more cups

Teenagers ... 4 or more cups

Adults ... 2 or more cups

RECOMMENDED

Milk products that are low in dairy fats:

Fortified skimmed (nonfat) milk and fortified skimmed milk powder • low-fat milk. The label on the container should show that the milk is fortified with vitamins A and D. The word "fortified" alone is not enough.

Buttermilk made from skimmed milk • yogurt made from skimmed milk • canned evaporated skimmed milk • cocoa made with low-fat milk.

Cheeses made from skimmed or partly skimmed milk, such as cottage cheese, creamed or uncreamed (uncreamed, preferably) • farmer's, baker's, or hoop cheese • mozzarella and sapsago cheeses.

AVOID OR USE SPARINGLY

Whole milk and whole milk products:

Chocolate milk • canned whole milk • ice cream • all creams including sour, half and half, whipped • whole milk yogurt.

Nondairy cream substitutes (usually contain coconut oil which is very high in saturated fat).

Cheeses made from cream or whole milk.

Butter.

5   FATS and OILS

(Polyunsaturated)

An individual allowance should include about 2–4 tablespoons daily (depending on how many calories you can afford) in the form of margarine, salad dressing, and shortening.

RECOMMENDED

AVOID OR USE SPARINGLY

Margarines, liquid oil shortenings, salad dressings and mayonnaise containing any of these polyunsaturated vegetable oils:

Corn oil • cottonseed oil • safflower oil • sesame seed oil • soybean oil • sunflower seed oil.

Margarines and other products high in polyunsaturates can usually be identified by their label which lists a recommended *liquid* vegetable oil as the *first* ingredient, and one or more partly hydrogenated vegetable oils as additional ingredients.

Diet margarines are low in calories because they are low in fat. Therefore it takes twice as much diet margarine to supply the polyunsaturates contained in a recommended margarine.

Solid fats and shortenings:

Butter • lard • salt pork fat • meat fat • completely hydrogenated margarines and vegetable shortenings • products containing coconut oil.

Peanut oil and olive oil may be used occasionally for flavor, but they are low in polyunsaturates and do not take the place of the recommended oils.

6 DESSERTS · BEVERAGES SNACKS · CONDIMENTS

The foods on this list are acceptable because they are low in saturated fat and cholesterol. If you have eaten your daily allowance from the first five lists, however, these foods will be in excess of your nutritional needs, and many of them also may exceed your calorie limits for maintaining a desirable weight. If you must limit calories, limit your portions of the foods on this list as well.

Moderation should be observed especially in the use of alcoholic drinks, ice milk, sherbet, sweets, and bottled drinks.

ACCEPTABLE

Low in calories or no calories
Fresh fruit and fruit canned without sugar • tea, coffee (no cream), cocoa powder • water ices • gelatin • fruit whip • puddings made with nonfat milk • sweets and bottled drinks made with artificial sweeteners • vinegar, mustard, ketchup, herbs, spices.

High in calories
Frozen or canned fruit with sugar added • jelly, jam, marmalade, honey • pure sugar candy such as gumdrops, hard candy, mint patties (not chocolate) • imitation ice cream made with safflower oil • cakes, pies, cookies, and puddings made with polyunsaturated fat in place of solid shortening • angel food cake • nuts, especially walnuts • non-hydrogenated peanut butter • bottled drinks • fruit drinks • ice milk • sherbet • wine, beer, whiskey.

AVOID OR USE SPARINGLY

Coconut and coconut oil • commercial cakes, pies, cookies, and mixes • frozen cream pies • commercially fried foods such as potato chips and other deep-fried snacks • whole milk puddings • chocolate pudding (high in cocoa butter and therefore high in saturated fat) • ice cream.

(Courtesy American Heart Association)

FOODS, FATS, CHOLESTEROL, AND CALORIES

The values shown are for servings of about 3⅓ ounces.

Foods	Saturated fats mgs.	Unsaturated fats mgs.	Cholesterol gms.	Calories
Meat, Fish, and Poultry				
Beef, lean	12	12	70	290
Chicken	8	14	60	110
Fish (fresh)	0	0	50–70	60–200
Lamb	12	9	70	135
Salmon	0	0	60	211
Shrimp	0	0	125	82
Tuna	0	0	60	146
Turkey	4	9	75	200
Veal	6	5	90	145
Cereals and dairy products				
Cornmeal	0	3	0	59
Cottage cheese	2	1	15	101
Rice	2	1	0	103
Wheat	2	8	0	109
Fats and oils				
Corn oil	10	81	0	900
Cottonseed oil	25	71	0	900
Margarine	18	61	65	733
Olive oil	11	83	0	900
Peanut oil	18	76	0	900
Safflower oil	8	87	0	900
Shortening, vegetable	23	72	0	733
Soybean oil	15	72	0	900

	Saturated fats mgs.	Unsaturated fats mgs.	Cholesterol gms.	Calories
Vegetables				
Asparagus	0	0	0	26
Lima beans	0	0	0	131
String beans	0	0	0	42
Beets	0	0	0	46
Broccoli	0	0	0	37
Brussels sprouts	0	0	0	58
Cabbage	0	0	0	29
Carrots	0	0	0	45
Celery	0	0	0	22
Corn	0	0	0	108
Cucumbers	0	0	0	14
Eggplant	0	0	0	28
Lettuce	0	0	0	18
Mushrooms	0	0	0	3
Olives	0	0	0	189
Onions	0	0	0	48
Peas	0	0	0	73
Potato chips	0	0	0	557
Potatoes, French fried	0	0	0	274
Potatoes, baked	0	0	0	94
Potatoes, mashed	0	0	0	115
Spinach	0	0	0	25
Squash	0	0	0	19
Tomatoes	0	0	0	23
Turnips	0	0	0	22
Fruit				
Apples	0	0	0	64
Apricots	0	0	0	56
Bananas	0	0	0	66
Cantaloupe	0	0	0	23
Grapefruit	0	0	0	29
Grapes	0	0	0	74
Oranges	0	0	0	36
Peaches	0	0	0	51
Pears	0	0	0	70

Pineapple	0	0	0	58
Plums	0	0	0	48
Strawberries	0	0	0	41
Watermelon	0	0	0	14

Courtesy National Institutes of Health, Washington, D.C.

100-CALORIE SERVINGS FOR COMMONLY USED FOODS

Cereals and breads

Biscuit or plain muffin	¾ medium
Bread, white, enriched	1½ slices
Corn flakes	1 cup
Crackers, saltines	6
Oatmeal, cooked	⅔ cup
Rice, white, cooked	½ cup
Roll, plain	⅚ medium
Wheat, puffed	2⅓ cups

Dairy products

Butter	1 tbsp.
Buttermilk	1⅙ cups
Cheese, Cheddar	⅞ oz.
Cheese, cottage	3⅔ oz.
Cream, heavy	2 tbsp.
Ice cream, plain	⅓ cup
Milk, whole	4⅘ oz.
Milk, nonfat solids	3½ tbsp.

Vegetables

Beans, lima, canned	⅔ cup
Beans, soup, green, canned	2⅔ cups
Broccoli, cooked	2¼ cups
Cabbage, shredded, raw	4⅙ cups
Carrots, raw	4¾ medium
Cauliflower, cooked	3⅓ cups
Celery, diced, raw	5½ cups
Corn, canned	¾ cup
Lettuce	1½ lb. head

Onion, cooked	1¼
Peas, green, canned	⅔ cup
Pepper, green, raw	5⅞ medium
Potato, white, baked	1 medium
Potato, white, mashed	⅔ cup
Potato, sweet, baked	½ medium
Spinach, cooked	2⅙ cups
Tomatoes, canned	2⅙ cups

Fats and oils

French dressing	1⅔ tbsp.
Mayonnaise	1 tbsp.
Salad oil	⅘ tbsp.

Fruit

Apple, raw	1⅓ medium
Apricot, canned	½ cup
Banana	1⅛ medium
Grapefruit juice, canned	1¹⁄₁₀ cups
Orange juice, fresh	⁹⁄₁₀ cup
Peaches or pears, canned	⅗ cup
Pineapple, canned, crushed	½ cup
Strawberries, raw	1⅚ cups

Meat, Fish, Poultry and Eggs, and Nuts

Bacon, cooked	2 slices
Beef, cooked	1 oz.
Chicken, breast, cooked	3⅘ oz.
Egg, whole	1¼
Frankfurter	⅘
Haddock, cooked	⅔ fillet
Ham, cooked	⁹⁄₁₀ oz.
Liver, beef, cooked	1¾ oz.
Luncheon meat	1⅕ oz.
Peanut butter	1¹⁄₁₀ tbsp.
Pork, cooked	1¹⁄₁₀ oz.
Tuna fish, canned	1⅘ oz.

Sugars and sweets

Carbonated beverage	8 oz.
Candy bar, chocolate	⅔ oz.
Cake, plain, iced	⅝ medium
Cookies, plain	⁹⁄₁₀ medium
Jellies	2 tbsp.
Pie, apple	½ medium
Syrup, corn	1¾ tbsp.
Sugar, white	6¼ tbsp.

Courtesy United States Department of Agriculture (*Food and Your Weight*).

CALORIE EXPENDITURES

Weight gain and weight loss depend not only upon caloric intake but also upon calories used. The body of course uses calories simply to maintain its functioning. Beyond that, energy needs—caloric expenditures—depend upon the kind of work and leisure time activities that a person engages in.

For convenience, various activities can be grouped into five general types, as they are in the following table. Because even for the same activity, there is some difference in caloric expenditure between people—some are more efficient in body actions—the table shows a range of even as much as 100 calories an hour.

Calories expended per hour	*Type of activity*
80–100	SEDENTARY: Includes such activities as reading, writing, watching TV or movies, sewing, playing cards, typing, general office work, other activities carried out while sitting that involve little or no movement of the arms.

110–160   LIGHT: Includes food preparation and cooking, dishwashing, dusting, washing small garments, ironing, personal care, slow walking, office work and activities done while standing and requiring some movement of the arms, and rapid typing, collating, etc., done while sitting.

170–240   MODERATE: Includes bed making, mopping, scrubbing, sweeping, polishing and waxing, light gardening, carpentry, moderately fast walking, other activities carried out while standing and calling for moderate arm movements, and any activity done while seated that involves fairly vigorous arm motions.

250–350   VIGOROUS: Includes heavy scrubbing and waxing, hanging out clothes, stripping beds, other heavy work, fast walking, gardening.

350–up   STRENUOUS: Includes swimming, tennis, running, bicycling, dancing, skiing, football. Actually, depending upon speed, running may call for calorie expenditures of from 800 to 1,300 an hour; swimming, 300 to 1,000; rowing, 1,000 to 1,500; cycling, 150 to 600. A very fast walk (5.3 miles an hour) may consume as many as 565 calories an hour.

Courtesy United States Department of Agriculture (*Food and Your Weight*).

DESIRABLE WEIGHTS

Desirable weights differ from average weights, and modern weight tables recognize the fact. For one thing, average people tend to become fat with time, and this is not desirable. Average weights reflect all weights, including the obese who make up the upper part of the average.

The following tables provide desirable weights, in pounds, for men and women, according to height and according to body frame, as ordinarily dressed indoors, with shoes.

Men

| Height (shoes on) | | Small frame | Medium frame | Large frame |
Feet	Inches			
5	2	116–125	124–133	131–142
5	3	119–128	127–136	133–144
5	4	122–132	130–140	137–149
5	5	126–136	134–144	141–153
5	6	129–139	137–147	145–157
5	7	133–143	141–151	149–162
5	8	136–147	145–160	153–166
5	9	140–151	149–160	157–170
5	10	144–155	153–164	161–175
5	11	148–164	157–168	165–180
6	0	152–164	161–173	169–185
6	1	157–169	166–178	174–190
6	2	163–175	171–184	179–196
6	3	168–180	176–189	184–202

Women

Feet	Inches	Small frame	Medium frame	Large frame
4	11	104–111	110–118	117–127
5	0	105–113	112–120	119–129
5	1	107–115	114–122	121–131
5	2	110–118	117–125	124–135
5	3	113–121	120–128	127–138
5	4	116–125	124–132	131–142
5	5	119–128	127–135	133–145

5	6	123–132	130–140	138–150
5	7	126–136	134–144	142–154
5	8	129–139	137–147	145–158
5	9	133–143	141–151	149–162
5	10	136–147	145–155	152–166
5	11	139–150	148–158	155–169

Courtesy Simon & Schuster (*Family Book of Preventive Medicine*, Miller & Galton).

THE PINCH TEST

The pinch, or skinfold, test is a relatively simple one for assessing actual fatness.

With thumb and forefinger, pick up a "pinch" of skin, at the waist, stomach, upper arm, buttocks, calf. Much of body fat is concentrated directly under the skin.

Generally, the layer beneath the skin—which is what you pick up with the pinch, since only fat, not muscle, pinches—should measure no more than half an inch. With your pinch, however, you are picking up a double thickness. Consequently, the thickness you pick up should measure no more than one inch. A fold greater than an inch indicates fatness.

A DICTIONARY OF MEDICAL TERMS

ADRENALIN (ad-ren'al-in). A secretion of the two small adrenal glands above the kidneys. The secretion, also called epinephrine, constricts the small blood vessels (arterioles), increases heart beat rate, and raises blood pressure.

ANEURYSM (an'u-rizm). A sac-like or spindle-shaped bulging of the wall of an artery or vein, resulting from weakening of the wall by disease or present as an abnormality at birth.

ANGINA PECTORIS (an'jin-ah pek'to-ris or an-ji'nah pek'to-ris). Chest pain caused by inadequate blood supply to the heart muscle, commonly the result of narrowing of the arteries feeding the heart muscle by atherosclerosis.

ANOXIA (an-ok'se-ah). Lack of oxygen. Most often occurs when blood supply to a part of the body is completely cut off. This leads to death of the tissue. For example, a part of the heart muscle may die when its blood (and therefore oxygen) supply is blocked by a clot in the artery supplying the area.

ANTIHYPERTENSIVE (an'te-hi-per-ten'siv) AGENT. A drug used to lower blood pressure.

ANXIETY (ang-zi'e-te). Feeling of apprehension, although no cause of the feeling is recognized.

AORTA (a-or'tah). The main trunk artery of the body. It begins at the base of the heart, receives blood from the heart's main pumping chamber (left ventricle). After arching up over the heart somewhat like the handle of a cane, it passes down through chest and abdomen in front of the spine. From the aorta branch off many arteries that carry blood to all areas of the body except the lungs, which get blood through other vessels coming directly from the heart.

APOPLEXY (ap'o-plek-se). Also called apoplectic stroke or stroke. A sudden shutoff of blood flow to a part of the brain as the result of blockage or rupture of an artery. It may first lead to loss of consciousness, sensation or voluntary movement, and may leave part of the body, often one side, temporarily or permanently paralyzed.

ARRHYTHMIA (ah-rith'me-ah). An abnormal heart beat rhythm.

ARTERIAL BLOOD (ar-te're-al). Blood that has picked up oxygen in the lungs, returns to the heart through the pulmonary veins, and then is pumped into the aorta and arteries to be carried to all body areas.

ARTERIOLES (ar-te're-ols). The smallest arterial vessels (about 1/125 inch in diameter). They pass blood from arteries to capillaries, the latter being vessels through which oxygen and nutrients can move into the tissues.

ARTERIOSCLEROSIS (ar-te're-o-skle-ro'sis). Hardening of the arteries. A broad term that includes various conditions causing artery walls to thicken, harden, lose elasticity. See *Atherosclerosis*.

ARTERY (ar'ter-e). A blood vessel transporting blood away from the heart to a body area.

ATHEROMA (ath-er-o'mah). A deposit of materials, including fatty substances, in the inner lining of an artery wall, characteristic of atherosclerosis.

ATHEROSCLEROSIS (ath'er-o-skle-ro'sis). A kind of arteriosclerosis in which the inner layer of the artery wall is made thick and irregular by deposits of fatty substances and other materials. The deposits, extending above the normal surface of the inner layer of the artery, decrease the diameter of the vessel's internal channel.

ATRIUM (a'tre-um). One of the heart's two upper chambers. Sometimes called auricle. The right atrium receives "used" or unoxygenated blood back from the body; the left atrium receives oxygenated blood from the lungs.

AUTONOMIC NERVOUS SYSTEM (aw-to-nom'ik). Also called the involuntary or vegetative nervous system. It regulates the functioning of organs and tissues not under voluntary control, including heart, glands, smooth muscles.

BLOOD PRESSURE. The pressure of blood in the arteries. The pressure when the heart muscle contracts (systole) is called systolic. Blood pressure when the heart muscle relaxes (diastole) between beats is called diastolic.

CALORIE (kal'o-re). Also called large or kilo-calorie. A unit that expresses food energy. It represents the amount of heat needed to raise the temperature of 1 kilogram of water 1 degree centigrade. A high calorie diet has a caloric value above the total daily energy requirement; a low calorie diet has a caloric value below the energy requirement.

CAPILLARIES (kap'i-lar-ez). Very narrow tubes that form a network between arterioles and veins. Their walls consist of just a single layer of cells through which oxygen and nutrients pass to the tissues and carbon dioxide and waste products pass from tissues into blood stream.

CARDIAC (kar'de-ak). Having to do with the heart. Also used to refer to anyone who has heart disease.

CARDIAC OUTPUT. The amount of blood pumped by the heart a minute.

CARDIOVASCULAR (kar'-de-o-vas'ku-lar). Having to do with the heart and blood vessels.

CARDIOVASCULAR-RENAL DISEASE (kar'de-o-vas'ku-lar re'nal). Disease involving heart, blood vessels, and kidneys.

CAROTID ARTERIES (kah-rot'id). The left and right common carotid arteries are the principal vessels supplying the head and neck. Each has two major branches, external and internal carotid.

CAROTID SINUS (kah-rot'id si'nus). A slight dilation at the point where the internal carotid artery branches from the common carotid artery. In the dilation, or carotid sinus, are nerve end organs sensitive to changes in blood pressure. In response to the changes, they change the heartbeat rate. Pressing on the carotid sinus can stimulate the nerves and cause a drop in blood pressure and faintness.

CEREBRAL VASCULAR ACCIDENT (ser'e-bral vas'ku-lar). Also called cerebrovascular accident, apoplectic stroke or stroke. A sudden interruption of blood supply to part of the brain.

CEREBROVASCULAR (ser'e-bro-vas'ku-lar). Having to do with the blood vessels in the brain.

CHEMOTHERAPY (ke-mo-ther'ah-pe). The treatment of disease by use of chemicals. Thus, chemotherapy of hypertension is the treatment of high blood pressure by drugs.

CHOLESTEROL (ko-les'ter-ol). A fatlike substance found in animal tissue. In blood tests, the normal level for Americans is considered to be between 180 and 230 milligrams of cholesterol for each 100 cubic centimeters of blood.

CIRCULATORY (ser'ku-lah-to-re). Having to do with the heart, blood vessels, and circulation of the blood.

COAGULATION (ko-ag-u-la'shun). Change from liquid to thickened or solid state. The formation of a clot.

COARCTATION OF THE AORTA (ko-ark-ta'shun of the a-or'ta). A narrowing or pressing together of the aorta, the main trunk artery.

COLLATERAL CIRCULATION (ko-lat'er-al ser'ku-la'shun). Circulation of the blood through nearby smaller vessels when a main vessel has been blocked.

CONGESTIVE (kon-jes'tiv) HEART FAILURE. When the heart loses some of its efficiency and is unable to pump out all the blood that returns to it, blood backs up in the veins leading to the heart. Congestion, or fluid accumulation, in lungs, legs, abdomen, or other parts of the body may result from the heart's failure to maintain satisfactory circulation.

CONSTRICTION (kon-strik'shun). Narrowing, as in "vaso-constriction," which is a narrowing of the internal diameter of blood vessels, caused by contraction of the muscular coat of the vessels.

CORONARY (kor'o-na-re) ARTERIES. The two arteries that branch off from the aorta and carry blood to the heart muscle.

CORONARY ATHEROSCLEROSIS (kor'o-na-re ath'er-o-skle-ro'sis). Commonly called coronary heart disease. A thickening by abnormal deposits of the inner layer of the walls of the coronary arteries carrying blood to the heart muscle. With the thickening, the internal channel of the arteries becomes narrowed and blood supply to the heart muscle is reduced.

CORONARY OCCLUSION (kor'o-na-re ok-klu'zhun). An obstruction, usually a blood clot, in a branch of a coronary artery. The obstruction impedes blood flow to some part of the heart muscle that dies because of lack of nourishment. Sometimes called a coronary heart attack, or heart attack.

CORONARY THROMBOSIS (kor'o-na-re throm-bo'sis). The development of a clot in a coronary artery branch. A form of coronary occlusion. See *Coronary Occlusion.*

DIASTOLE (di-as'to-le). The period of relaxation of the heart between beats.

DIGITALIS (dig-e-ta'lis). A drug obtained from the leaves of the foxglove plant that strengthens the contraction of the heart muscle, slows the contraction rate, and by improving heart efficiency may lead to the elimination of excess fluid from body tissues.

DILATION (di-la'shun). Stretching or enlargement of heart or blood vessels.

DIURESIS (di-u-re'sis). Increased excretion of urine.

DIURETIC (di-u-ret'ik). A drug that promotes excretion of urine.

DYSPNEA (disp-ne'ah). Difficult or labored breathing.

EDEMA (e-de'mah). Swelling due to abnormal amounts of fluid retained in the body tissues.

EKG. See *Electrocardiogram.*

ELECTROCARDIOGRAM (e-lek'tro-kar'de-o-gram). Often called EKG or ECG. A graphic record of electric currents produced by the heart.

ELECTROCARDIOGRAPH (e-lek'tro-kar'de-o-graf). An instrument for recording the electric currents produced by the heart.

ELECTROLYTE (e-lek'tro-lite). Any substance, such as sodium or potassium, which in solution can conduct electricity by means of its atoms or groups of atoms and in the process is broken down into positively and negatively charged particles.

EMBOLISM (em'bo-lizm). The obstruction of a blood vessel by a clot or other material carried in the blood stream from another site.

EMBOLUS (em'bo-lus). A blood clot—or another substance such as fat or air—inside a blood vessel that is transported in the blood stream to a smaller vessel and there becomes an obstruction to circulation.

EPIDEMIOLOGY (ep'e-de-me-ol'o-je). A science concerned with factors determining the frequency and distribution of disease.

EPINEPHRINE (ep-e-nef'rin). A secretion of the adrenal glands atop the kidneys, also called adrenalin. It constricts arterioles and raises blood pressure and is classified as a vasoconstrictor or vasopressor substance.

ESSENTIAL HYPERTENSION (hi-per-ten'shun). Commonly known as high blood pressure; sometimes called primary hypertension; an elevated pressure not caused by kidney or other evident disease.

EYEGROUND (i'ground). The inside of the back part of the eye seen through the pupil. Also called the fundus of the eye. An examination of the eyeground is one means of noting changes in blood vessels.

FUNDUS OF THE EYE (fun'dus). See *Eyeground.*

GANGLION (gang'gle-on). A collection of nerve cells serving as a nerve center.

GANGLIONIC BLOCKING AGENT (gang-gle-on'ik). A drug that interrupts transmission of nerve impulses at the nerve centers (ganglia). Such a drug may be used for high blood pressure.

HEMIPLEGIA (hem-e-ple'je-ah). Paralysis of one side of the body as the result of damage to the opposite side of the brain. Nerves cross in the brain so that one side of the brain controls the opposite arm and leg. Such paralysis is sometimes caused by a blood clot or hemorrhage in a brain blood vessel. See *Stroke*.

HEMORRHAGE (hem'or-ij). Escape of blood from a blood vessel. In external hemorrhage, blood is lost from the body; in internal hemorrhage, blood passes into tissues surrounding the ruptured blood vessel.

HYPERTENSION (hi-per-ten'shun). Commonly called high blood pressure. May be *essential* hypertension, without known cause, or *secondary* hypertension, stemming from kidney or other disease.

HYPOTENSION (hi-po-ten'shun). Commonly called low blood pressure. Blood pressure below the normal range.

INFARCT (in'farkt). An area of tissue damaged or dead as a result of receiving insufficient blood. As used in the phrase "myocardial infarct" it refers to a heart muscle area damaged or killed by insufficient blood flow through a coronary artery that normally supplies the area.

INSUFFICIENCY (in-suh-fish'en-se). Incompetency. In the term "myocardial insufficiency," it means inability of the heart to pump normally.

INTIMA (in'te-mah). The innermost layer of a blood vessel.

ISCHEMIA (is-ke'me-ah). A localized and usually temporary shortage of blood in some part of the body that may be caused by a constriction or obstruction in a blood vessel supplying that part.

LIPID (lip'id). Fat.

MALIGNANT HYPERTENSION (mah-lig'nant hi-per-ten'shun). Severe high blood pressure that can run a rapid course.

METABOLISM (me-tab'o-lizm). All the chemical changes that take place within the body.

MONO-UNSATURATED FAT (mon-o-un-sat'u-rat-ed). A fat so chemically constructed that it can absorb additional hydrogen but not as much hydrogen as a polyunsaturated fat. Mono-unsaturated fats in the diet have little effect on cholesterol levels in the blood. Olive oil is an example of such a fat.

MORBIDITY (mor-bid'i-te) RATE. The ratio of the number of cases of a disease to the number of healthy people in a given population for a year or other period of time. The term "morbidity" includes two concepts: (1) incidence, or the number of new cases of a disease in a given population during a set period of time; (2) prevalence, the number of cases of a disease existing in a given population at a particular moment in time.

MORTALITY (mor-tal'i-te) RATE. Various mortality rate classifications are used. The *crude* mortality rate, or crude death rate, is the ratio of total deaths to total population during a year or other period of time. *Age-adjusted* mortality rates are death rates that have been standardized for age to allow comparisons between different populations or within the same population at various intervals of time. Age-specific death rates of the populations under comparison are applied to a population arbitrarily selected as standard, to establish what would be the crude death rate in the standard population if it were exposed first to the rates of one population and to those of the other. An *age-specific* death rate is the ratio of deaths in a specific age group to the population of the same age group during a year or other period of time. *Cause-specific* death rate is the ratio of mortality from a specific cause to total population in a year or other period of time.

MYOCARDIAL INFARCTION (mi-o-kar'de-al in-fark'shun). Damage or death of an area of the heart muscle (myocardium) caused by reduced blood supply reaching the area.

MYOCARDIAL INSUFFICIENCY (mi-o-kar'de-al). Inability of the heart muscle (myocardium) to maintain normal circulation. See *Congestive Heart Failure.*

MYOCARDIUM (mi-o-kar'de-um). The muscular wall of the heart.

NEUROGENIC (nu-ro-jen'ik). Originating in the nervous system.

NITROGLYCERIN (ni-tro-glis'er-in). A vasodilator drug that relaxes the muscles in blood vessels. Often used to relieve or help prevent attacks of angina pectoris.

NORADRENALIN (nor-ad-ren'ah-lin). A compound, also called norepinephrine and levarterenol, which raises blood pressure by constricting small blood vessels.

NOREPINEPHRINE (nor'ep-e-nef'rin). See *Noradrenalin.*

NORMOTENSIVE (nor-mo-ten'siv). Characterized by normal blood pressure.

PALPITATION (pal-pi-ta'shun). A fluttering of the heart or abnormal rhythm or rate of the heart sensed by an individual himself.

PARAPLEGIA (par-ah-ple'je-ah). Loss of motion and sensation in legs and lower part of body. Most often this is due to spinal cord damage but sometimes may result from a blood clot or hemorrhage in an artery carrying blood to the spinal cord.

PARASYMPATHETIC NERVOUS SYSTEM (par'ah-sim-path-thet'ik). A part of the involuntary, or autonomic, nervous system. The parasympathetic nerves carry impulses that contract the pupils of the eyes, slow the heart rate, and produce other involuntary reactions.

PATHOGENESIS (path-o-jen'e-sis). The events leading to the development of disease.

PERIPHERAL RESISTANCE (peh-rif'er-al). The resistance to blood flow from arteries to veins offered by the arterioles and capillaries. Increased peripheral resistance raises blood pressure.

POLYUNSATURATED FAT (pol-e-un-sat'u-rat-ed). A fat so made up chemically that it can absorb additional hydrogen. Polyunsaturated fats are usually liquid oils of vegetable origin, such as corn or safflower oil. A diet with high polyunsaturated fat content tends to lower cholesterol levels in the blood. See *Mono-unsaturated fat.*

PRESSOR (pres'or). A substance that raises blood pressure and speeds the heartbeat.

PREVALENCE (prev'ah-lense). The number of cases of a disease in a given population at a specific time.

PRIMARY HYPERTENSION (hi-per-ten'shun). Also called essential hypertension and commonly known as high blood pressure. An elevated pressure not related to kidney or other apparent disease.

PROPHYLAXIS (pro-fi-lak'sis). Preventive treatment.

PSYCHOSOMATIC (si-ko-so-mat'ik). Having to do with the influence of mind and emotions upon the functions of the body, especially in terms of disease.

PSYCHOTHERAPY (si-ko-ther'ah-pe). The treatment of disorders through suggestion, persuasion, education, counseling, or psychoanalysis.

PULMONARY ARTERY (pul-mo-na-re). The large artery that carries used unoxygenated blood from the heart to the lungs; it is the only artery that carries unoxygenated blood.

PULSE (pulse). The expansion and contraction of an artery, which may be felt with the finger at the wrist or elsewhere. The artery contractions correspond to contractions of the heart and so are indications of heartbeat.

PULSE PRESSURE (pulse). The difference between the blood pressure in the arteries when the heart contracts (systole) and when it relaxes (diastole). Thus, an individual with a systolic pressure of 140 and a diastolic pressure of 90 (140/90) has a pulse pressure of 50 (140–90).

RENAL (re'nal). Having to do with the kidney.

RENAL CIRCULATION (re'nal). The circulation of blood through the kidneys.

RENAL HYPERTENSION (re'nal hi-per-ten'shun). High blood pressure caused by damage to or disease of the kidneys.

SATURATED FAT (sat'u-rat-ed). A fat so made up chemically that it can absorb no more hydrogen. Saturated fats are usually solid fats of animal origin such as the fats in meat, milk, butter. A diet high in saturated fats tends to raise cholesterol levels in the blood.

SCLEROSIS (skle-ro'-sis). Hardening, usually due to accumulation of fibrous material.

SECONDARY HYPERTENSION (hi-per-ten'shun). Elevated blood pressure caused by—therefore, secondary to—a specific disease.

Appendix

SEDATIVE (sed'ah-tiv). A drug that depresses activity of the central
nervous system and thus has a calming effect.

SERUM (se'rum). The fluid portion of blood remaining after cellular
blood elements have been removed by coagulation. Serum differs
from plasma, which is the cell-free liquid portion of uncoagulated
blood.

SIGN. Any objective evidence of a disease. See *Symptom*.

SODIUM (so'de-um). A mineral found in nearly all plant and animal
tissue and essential to life. Table salt is sodium chloride, nearly half
sodium. In hypertension and some types of heart disease, excess
sodium and water may be retained in the body.

SPHYGMOMANOMETER (sfig'mo-mah-nom'e-ter). An instrument
for measuring blood pressure in the arteries.

STENOSIS (ste-no'sis). A narrowing.

STETHOSCOPE (steth'o-skōp). An instrument for listening to sounds
within the body.

STROKE (strōk). Also called apoplectic stroke, cerebrovascular accident, or cerebral vascular accident. The result of impeded blood supply to some part of the brain that may be caused by (1) a blood
clot forming in the vessel (cerebral thrombosis); (2) a rupture of a
blood vessel wall and escape of blood into the brain area nearby
(cerebral hemorrhage); (3) a clot or other material from elsewhere
in the circulatory system that flows to the brain and obstructs a brain
vessel (cerebral embolism); (4) pressure on a blood vessel, as by a
tumor.

SYMPATHECTOMY (sim-pah-thek'to-me). Surgery that interrupts
some part of the sympathetic nervous system. The sympathetic
nervous system is part of the autonomic, or involuntary, nervous
system and regulates such tissues as glands, heart, and smooth
muscles. When the interruption is achieved with drugs, it is called
a chemical sympathectomy.

SYMPATHETIC NERVOUS SYSTEM (sim-pah-thet'ik). A part of the
involuntary, or autonomic, nervous system that regulates such tissues
as glands, heart and smooth muscles not under voluntary control.
See also *Parasympathetic Nervous System*.

SYMPTOM (simp'tum). Any subjective evidence of a patient's condition. See also *Sign*.

SYNCOPE (sin'ko-pe). A faint. One cause is insufficient blood supply
to the brain.

SYNDROME (sin'drom). A set of symptoms that occur together and
are given a name to indicate the combination.

SYSTOLE (sis'to-le). The period of contraction of the heart.

TACHYCARDIA (tak-e-kar'de-ah). Abnormally fast heart rate, generally anything greater than 100 beats a minute.

TOXEMIA (toks-e'me-ah). The condition produced by poisonous substances in the blood.

TOXIC (tok'sik). Having to do with poison.

UREMIA (u-re'me-ah). Excess in the blood of waste materials normally excreted by the kidneys in the urine.

VASOCONSTRICTOR (vas'o-kon-strik'tor). Vasoconstrictor nerves are those in the involuntary, or autonomic, system which, when stimulated, cause arteriole muscles to contract, thus narrowing the arterioles, increasing their resistance to blood flow, and raising blood pressure. Chemical substances that contract the arteriole muscles are called vasoconstrictor agents, or vasopressors. One example is adrenalin, or epinephrine.

VASODILATOR (vas'o-di-lat'or). Vasodilator nerves are those in the involuntary, or autonomic, system which, when stimulated, cause arteriole muscles to relax, enlarging the arteriole passage, reducing resistance to blood flow, and lowering blood pressure. Vasodilator agents are chemicals that cause relaxation of arteriole muscles. Nitroglycerin is one example.

VASO-INHIBITOR (vas'o-in-hib'i-tor). A drug that inhibits action of the vasomotor nerves and thus causes arteriole muscles to relax, the arteriole passage to enlarge, and blood pressure to be lowered.

VASOPRESSOR (vas-o-pres'or). A drug that contracts muscles of the arterioles, narrowing the arteriole passage and raising blood pressure. Such a substance also is called a vasoconstrictor. One example is adrenalin, or epinephrine.

VEIN (vain). A vessel that carries blood from a part of the body back to the heart. All veins conduct unoxygenated, or used blood, except the pulmonary veins, which carry freshly oxygenated blood from the lungs back to the heart.

VENA CAVA (ve'nah ka'vah). The superior vena cava is a large vein carrying blood from the head, neck, and thorax to the heart. The inferior vena cava is a large vein carrying blood from the lower part of the body to the heart.

VENOUS BLOOD (ve'nus). Blood carried by the veins from all parts of the body back to the heart to be pumped to the lungs where it is oxygenated.

VENTRICLE (ven'tri-kil). One of the two lower chambers of the heart. The left ventricle pumps oxygenated blood through the aorta and other arteries to the body. The right ventricle pumps unoxygenated blood through the pulmonary artery to the lungs.

VENULE (ven'ul). A very small vein.

ADDITIONAL BACKGROUND SOURCES

Chapter 1:

Hospital Practice, 9/71.
Bulletin of New York Academy of Medicine, vol. 45, p. 1306 (1969).
Conference, University of Southern California, 5/25/70.
World Health Organization report in *Medical Tribune,* 12/15/71.
Editorial, *Journal of the American Medical Association,* 11/15/71.
Lasker Award Lecture, *ibid.*
"Comprehensive Treatment of Essential Hypertension—Why, When, How,"
by Jeremiah Stamler, M.D., in *Monographs on Hypertension,* 10/70.
"Hypertension: The Great Untreated Disease," editorial, *Medical Tribune,*
2/3/71.
"Facts on the Major Killing and Crippling Diseases in the United States,"
compiled by the National Health Education Committee, Inc., 866 United
Nations Plaza, New York, N.Y., 10017.

Chapter 2:

"Heart Facts, 1972," The American Heart Association.
"Primary Prevention of Hypertension," Report of Intersociety Commission
for Heart Disease Resources, *Circulation,* July 1970.
"Resources for the Management of Emergencies in Hypertension," Report
of Intersociety Commission for Heart Disease Resources, *Circulation,* March
1971.
"Heart in Industry," a newsletter to promote prevention of heart disease,
American Heart Association, Fall 1971.
Freedom from Heart Attacks, Benjamin F. Miller and Lawrence Galton
(Simon & Schuster, 1972).
The Family Book of Preventive Medicine, Benjamin F. Miller and Lawrence
Galton (Simon & Schuster, 1971).
See Also references for Chapter 1.

Chapter 3:

New York Academy of Sciences, vol. 149, p. 1038 (1968).
Journal of Chronic Diseases, vol. 22, p. 515.
Pathogenesis of Coronary Artery Disease, M. Friedman, M.D., New York:
McGraw-Hill, 1969.
"Arteriosclerosis," Report by National Heart and Lung Institute Task Force
on Arteriosclerosis, June 1971.

Chapter 4:

The Heart and Circulation, copyright 1965 by the Federation of American Societies for Experimental Biology.
Public Health Service study of 1966.
U.S. Air Force study: "Personality and Emotional Stress in Essential Hypertension in Man," Drs. Robert E. Harris and Ralph P. Forsyth, Cardiovascular Research Institute, University of California, San Francisco.
Intersociety Commission for Heart Disease Resources.
"Patterns in Hypertension," *Journal of the American Medical Association,* 9/7/70.
"Elevated Blood Pressure Levels in Adolescents," *Journal of the American Medical Association,* 9/15/69.
"Poll on Medical Practice, Hypertension," *Modern Medicine,* 8/10/70.

Chapter 5:

National Institutes of Health booklet no. 1714, *Hypertension.*
World Health Organization press release, 3/22/72.
Psychosomatic Medicine, vol. 32, p. 1, 1970.
U.S. Air Force study (cited in previous chapter notes).
Psychosomatic Specificity, vol. 1, University of Chicago Press, 1968.

Chapter 6:

Office Evaluation of the Hypertensive Patient, published by the American Heart Association.
New York State Journal of Medicine, 8/15/65.
Hahnemann Symposium on Hypertension, 12/71.
"The Hypertensive Evaluation," *American Family Physician,* 2/72.

Chapter 7:

Family Book of Preventive Medicine, by B. F. Miller and Lawrence Galton (Simon & Schuster, 1971).
Modern Medicine, Symposium on Hypertension, 3/20/72, p. 81.
Harvard study at Camp Lejeune, North Carolina, by Dr. George V. Mann.
"The Health Consequences of Smoking," a report of the Surgeon General: 1971.

Chapter 8:

"Treatment of Arterial Hypertension," *Modern Medicine,* 8/10/70.
"Drug Therapy of Essential Hypertension," *Modern Medicine,* 11/29/71.
"The Chemotherapy of Hypertension," *Journal of the American Medical Association,* 11/15/71.
"Optimum Therapy for Essential Hypertension," *American Family Physician,* 7/6/72.
"Medical Treatment of Chronic Hypertension," *Modern Concepts of Cardiovascular Disease,* American Heart Association, 4/71.

Chapter 9:

Modern Medicine, 11/29/71.
"Symposium on Hypertension," *American Journal of Medicine*, 5/72.
See also references for Chapter 8.

Chapter 11:

"Join the Campaign to Conquer High Blood Pressure," Lawrence Galton, *The Reader's Digest*, 2/73.
"Heart Attack and Stroke in Essential Hypertension: The Renin Factor," Hans R. Brunner and John H. Laragh, Hahnemann Symposium.
"Hypertension in the Inner City," Frank A. Finnerty, Jr., M.D., *American Family Physician*, 3/72.
"The New Mystery—Maybe Miracle—Drug," Lawrence Galton, *The New York Times Magazine*, 12/5/71.

Index

Adolescents, incidence of hypertension among, 51–52
Adrenal glands
  disorders of. *See* Aldosteronism; Pheochromocytoma
  effects of smoking on, 104
Adrenalin. *See* Epinephrine
Age
  heart attacks and, 3, 4, 5
  hypertension and, 50–52
  strokes and, 4–5
Alabama University Medical School, follow-up study conducted by, 50, 71–72
Aldosterone, 87, 89
Aldosteronism
  as cause of hypertension, 87
  detection of, 91
  primary, 87, 123
Allopurinol, 126
Alpha methyl norepinephrine, 115
Alpha-methyldopa. *See* Methyldopa
American Heart Association, 49–50
  on emotions and high blood pressure, 77
Amphetamines, 96
Anger, blood pressure and, 49
Angina pectoris, 16
  definition of, 15
  description of attack of, 38–39
  hypertension and, 6
  overweight as factor in, 20–21
  relationship to heart disease, 15
Aorta, coarctation of the, 63, 83–84, 91
  detection of, 91, 120
  testing for, 120
Arteries, 24–26
  brain, hypertension and, 37
  hardening of. *See* Atherosclerosis
  pulmonary, 42
Arterioles, 26–27, 30, 34, 111, 112
Aspirin, 125, 142
Atherosclerosis, 133
  causes of, 40–42

cholesterol and, 97–98
control of, 97
earliest indication of, 37–38
hypertension and, 6, 37, 97, 133
laboratory experiments concerning, 44–45
overweight and, 41
Pittsburgh University study of lesions, 43
plaque of, 38, 39, 41
smoking as factor in, 41
Atlanta, Georgia, hypertension study, 8
Autonomic nervous system, 32, 34

Baldwin County, Georgia, hypertension study, 8
Baltimore City Hospital, premature ventricular contraction study, 145
Bantu, 40
Baroreceptors, 30–31, 34
Baylor University Medical School, 90
Benign hypertension, 13, 61–62
Bergen County, New Jersey, hypertension control program, 151–52
Bible, stroke incidents cited in the, 16
Blacks, hypertension and, 54–55, 72–74
Blood pressure
  cause of, 23
  control of, 29
    drugs and, 115
  danger point, 56–57
  definition of, 23
  diastolic, 19, 28, 29, 57, 58, 59
  effect of exercise on, 101–3
  hormones and, 32, 34
  ideal, 59
  life expectancy and, 132
  measurement of, 17–18, 27–29
    home, 124
  normal, 28